OCCUPATIONAL THERAPY INTERVENTION RESOURCE MANUAL

A Guide for Occupation-Based Practice

OCCUPATIONAL THERAPY INTERVENTION RESOURCE MANUAL

A Guide for Occupation-Based Practice

Denise Chisholm, MS, OTR/L
Assistant Professor, University of Pittsburgh

Cathy Dolhi, MS, OTR/L, FAOTA
Assistant Professor, Chatham College

Jodi Schreiber, MS, OTR/L
Independent Consultant

THOMSON

DELMAR LEARNING

Australia Canada Mexico Singapore Spain United Kingdom United States

THOMSON

DELMAR LEARNING

Occupational Therapy Intervention Resource Manual: A Guide for Occupation-Based Practice
Denise Chisholm, Cathy Dolhi, and Jodi Schreiber

Vice President, Health Care Business Unit:
William Brottmiller

Editorial Director:
Cathy L. Esperti

Acquisitions Editor:
Kalen Conerly

Developmental Editor:
Maria D'Angelico

Marketing Director:
Jennifer McAvey

Channel Manager:
Lisa Osgood

Marketing Coordinator:
Chris Manion

Art/Design Specialist:
Jay Purcell

Project Editor:
Natalie Wager

Production Coordinator:
Bridget Lulay

Library of Congress Cataloging-in-Publication Data
Chisholm, Denise.
    Occupational therapy intervention resource manual: a guide for occupation-based practice / Denise Chisholm, Cathy Dolhi,
    Jodi Schreiber.—1st ed.
      p. ; cm.
    Includes bibliographical references.
      ISBN 1-4018-1536-7
    1. Occupational therapy.
    [DNLM: 1. Occupational Therapy—Handbooks. 2. Patient Care Planning—Handbooks.
    3. Professional Practice—Handbooks. WB 39 C542o 2004]
    I. Dolhi, Cathy II. Schreiber, Jodi. III. Title.
      RM735.C486 2004
      615.8'515—dc22

2003016406
ISBN 1-4018-1536-7

Notice to the Reader

Publisher does not warrant or guarantee any of the products described herein or perform any independent analysis in connection with any of the product information contained herein. Publisher does not assume, and expressly disclaims, any obligation to obtain and include information other than that provided to it by the manufacturer.

The reader is expressly warned to consider and adopt all safety precautions that might be indicated by the activities described herein and to avoid all potential hazards. By following the instructions contained herein, the reader willingly assumes all risks in connection with such instructions.

The publisher makes no representations or warranties of any kind, including but not limited to the warranties of fitness for particular purpose or merchantability, nor are any such representations implied with respect to the material set forth herein, and the publisher takes no responsibility with respect to such material. The publisher shall not be liable for any special, consequential, or exemplary damages resulting, in whole or part, from the reader's use of, or reliance upon, this material.

CONTENTS

PREFACE

Occupational therapy practitioners have been strongly encouraged to refocus their attention on occupation and its use as intervention. The transition from a medical model and the reductionistic care associated with it to occupation-based practice which emphasizes a client-centered approach has strengthened the profession's position within health care and reaffirmed the domain of occupational therapy. This paradigm shift requires occupational therapy practitioners to develop intervention programs that are individualized, meaningful, and oriented toward the clients' occupations and occupational performance. Despite valuing the concepts associated with occupation-based practice, the reality for occupational therapists, occupational therapy assistants, and occupational therapy students is that providing occupation-based interventions is often perceived and experienced as a challenge.

This manual is the culmination of a series of workshops designed and presented by the authors over the past four years. The audiences for these workshops have included occupational therapists, occupational therapy assistants, and occupational therapy students with varying degrees of clinical experience who represented a wide range of practice settings. While their differences have been many, the feedback from the more than 300 individuals who have participated in the workshops has been consistent. They have reported that the information and perspective is timely and clinically relevant; the topic is supported by background information that is significant to practice; and the information is applicable to their current clinical practice and/or would be a valuable resource for the future.

During our over 50 years of combined clinical experience, we have had the opportunity to be actively involved in the provision of occupational therapy services in many capacities including direct service provider, staff supervisor, fieldwork educator, manager, educator, and consultant. These opportunities have been pursued in a variety of physical medicine and mental health practice settings including acute care, inpatient rehabilitation, skilled nursing, long-term care, assisted living, outpatient, home care, and academia. Throughout these experiences, our belief in the use of occupation as the core of occupational therapy intervention and as a motivational force for helping people to achieve their goals has remained steadfast. Our ongoing study and use of occupation in our clinical and academic practices has helped to strengthen our understanding and appreciation of the value and efficacy of occupation-based intervention.

ORGANIZATION AND USE OF THIS MANUAL

This manual is designed as a workbook to strengthen your understanding of occupation as the hallmark of occupational therapy intervention and to assist you in determining how intervention grounded in occupation may be best integrated into your clinical practice. Some of the pages are designed to be copied and used as worksheets. Whether you are a student engaged in the study of occupational therapy, or an experienced practitioner who is exploring options for enhancing the use of occupation-based interventions in your clinical practice, we hope that you will find this manual to be an important tool in facilitating occupation-based practice.

We have incorporated the terms "you" and "your" throughout this manual. The strategic use of these possessive pronouns is intended to encourage *you* to consider, throughout your reading and completion of the learning exercises, how the information can be applied to *your* practice. In addition, we hope that personalizing the content will facilitate the integration of the concepts into your clinical practice habit patterns.

The focus of this manual is three-fold. First, in addition to providing background information and reference materials related to occupation-based practice, you will have the opportunity to engage in a variety of learning exercises. These learning exercises are designed to "check your thinking"—that is, we hope that the exercises will enhance your understanding of occupation-based practice and assist you in identifying how occupation is and can be included in your clinical practice. Empty boxes have been included throughout the manual to allow you to write your ideas directly in the book. Second, we have provided you with a section of practical "tried and true" ideas for ways to maximize your ability to include occupation-based interventions in your clinical practice, plus guidance for obtaining evidence related to occupation-based interventions. Finally, we provide clinical scenarios depicting common practice situations that illustrate how occupation-based practice can be incorporated into a client's occupational therapy intervention plan. The clinical scenarios represent clients across the lifespan with a variety of conditions within different practice settings. We hope that your clinical reasoning skills will be enhanced through the identification, development, and planning of occupational therapy intervention plans based on occupation.

We anticipate that this manual will also be useful in facilitating classroom and mentorship discussions, providing insight into your own clinical practice, and stimulating problem-solving strategies that will enhance your ability to plan and implement occupation-based intervention. You are encouraged to use the learning exercises and the practice analysis with other practitioners and students to promote and facilitate the use of occupation-based interventions in your and their respective practices. You may discover that the learning exercises will stimulate dialogue and debate about occupation-based practice. These ongoing conversations can contribute to your clinical reasoning, your professional growth as an occupational therapy practitioner, and your commitment to being a life-long learner. The appendices may be reproduced and used for learning purposes; however, the reproducible sections may not be reprinted or resyndicated in whole or in part as a reproducible handout book or collection, or for any other purpose without the written permission of the publisher.

This manual is not intended to recommend nor prescribe occupational therapy interventions for any specific client or client population. All of the clinical scenarios are fictitious and the occupational profile and analysis of occupational performance, sample interventions, and intervention sessions associated with the clinical scenarios should not be interpreted as representing best practice. The clinical scenarios are provided for the sole purpose of illustrating the concepts of occupation-based practice.

It is important to note that this manual has come to fruition at a time when the language of the profession is undergoing a significant transition. "Uniform Terminology for Occupational Therapy—Third Edition," which provided an outline of the domain of concern of occupational therapy and created common terminology for the profession, was rescinded by the Representative Assembly of the American Occupational Therapy Association in May, 2002. "The Occupational Therapy Practice Framework: Domain and Process" has replaced this document. We have attempted to integrate information from both documents in an effort to appropriately reflect the domain of concern of occupational therapy while using terminology and concepts that are familiar to both current and future practitioners and students. We strongly encourage you to obtain and become familiar with "The Occupational Therapy Practice Framework: Domain and Process" and incorporate the concepts, process, and terminology into your practice.

ACKNOWLEDGMENTS

We would like to express our sincere gratitude and appreciation to our colleagues and mentors who have provided significant support and feedback for this project; the countless students and clinicians who have contributed to and challenged our thinking; and the expert practitioners who created the clinical scenarios. Without the valuable input from all of these individuals, this workbook would have remained an "idea"—never finding its way to the page. Finally, we would like to acknowledge and thank our families without whom our respective occupations would be meaningless!

We hope that this manual will be a useful tool to you as you embark on or continue your journey toward providing occupational therapy services centered in occupation.

Contributors

Dave Baldwin, BS, OTR/L
Patty Chambers, OTR/L
Carolyn M. Gatty, MS, OTR/L, CEAS
Stephen B. Kern, MS, OTR/L, FAOTA
Mary Lou (Kieshauer) Leibold, MS, OTR/L
Lynne "Cricket" T. Rizzo, MS, OTR/L, ATP
Joyce Salls, MS, OTR/L, BCP
Debby A. Sanchioli, MS, OTR/L
Leslie Sober, MOT, OTR/L
Pamela E. Toto, MS, OTR/L, BCG
Suzanne M. Trump, M.Div., MA, OTR/L
Michele Yotz, OTR/L

Reviewers

Shari Tayar, MA, OTR/L
Assistant Professor and Academic Fieldwork Coordinator
Physical and Occupational Therapy
Idaho State University
Pocatello, ID

Karen P. Funk, MA, OTR
Clinical Assistant Professor
Occupational Therapy Department
University of Texas at El Paso
El Paso, TX

Becky Roose MS, OTR/L
Private Practice
West Des Moines, IA

Catherine Emery, MS, OTR/L, BCN
Interim Dean of Enrollment Management
Occupational Therapy Department
Alvernia College
Lancaster, PA

Lisa Link Melville, MS, OTR/L
Clinical Assistant Professor, and Coordinator of Fieldwork Education and
Professional Development
Occupational Therapy Department
Medical College of Ohio
Toledo, OH

Wendy Prabst
Courtney St. Rehabilitation Clinic
Rhinelander, WI

Peter Scotto, OTR/L
Owner of Advanced Therapy
Slingerlands, NY

CHAPTER 1

Occupation-Based Practice

Learning Objectives

After reading this chapter, you should be able to do the following:

1. Describe occupation and its relevance to occupational therapy.
2. Describe occupation-based practice.
3. Identify resources that support the use of occupation-based practice.

Key Terms and Concepts

occupation
occupation-based practice

INTRODUCTION

Occupational therapy practitioners and students recognize the importance of engaging clients in meaningful and relevant occupations to facilitate health and wellness. However, as individuals, and over the years as a profession, we have struggled to define **occupation** and to articulate the value of using occupation in occupational therapy practice. Many of the leaders in our profession have attempted to define and clarify occupation (Baum & Baptiste, 2002; Clark et al., 1991; Law, Polatajko, Baptiste, & Townsend, 1997). Phrases such as "ordinary and familiar things that people do every day" (Clark et al., 1991, p. 300), "groups of activities and tasks of everyday life" (Law et al., 1997, p. 34), "everything people do to occupy himself or herself" (Law et al., 1997, p. 34), "the interaction of the individual with his or her self-directed life activities" (Baum & Baptiste, 2002, p. 11), and "as necessary to life as food and drink" (Dunton as cited in Peloquin, 1991, p. 734) have been used in an attempt to capture the meaning of occupation. The "Occupational Therapy Practice Framework: Domain and Process" (Framework) (American Occupational Therapy Association [AOTA], 2002) describes occupations as "having unique meaning and purpose in a person's life," "being central to a person's identity and competence," and influencing "how one spends time and makes decisions." The Framework (AOTA, 2002) defines occupation as:

> [A]ctivities . . . of everyday life, named, organized, and given value and meaning by individuals and a culture. Occupation is everything people do to occupy themselves, including looking after themselves, . . . enjoying life, . . . and contributing to the social and economic fabric of their communities . . . . (Law, Polatajko, Baptiste, & Townsend as cited in AOTA, 2002, p. 610)

Areas of occupation are categorized in the Framework (AOTA, 2002) as activities of daily living, instrumental activities of daily living, education, work, play, leisure, and social participation.

Baum and Baptiste (2002) identify the challenge for occupational therapy practitioners as moving beyond establishing goals to achieve functional independence to a model that makes the client's need for occupation central to the occupational therapy process with participation as the outcome. When practitioners include the client's meaningful and relevant occupations in their client's occupational therapy intervention plan, they are departing from a medical model approach and are progressing toward an **occupation-based practice** model.

RESOURCES

Literature and resources are available to occupational therapy practitioners that support the need for and the use of occupation-based practice. Table 1-1 provides a list of documents that you may find useful when describing the scope and benefit of

Table 1-1 Resources That Support Occupation-Based Practice.

DOCUMENT	QUOTATION
American Occupational Therapy Association. (1979). The philosophical base of occupational therapy. *American Journal of Occupational Therapy, 33,* 785.	Occupational therapy is based on the belief that purposeful activity (occupation), including its interpersonal and environmental components, may be used to prevent and mediate dysfunction, and to elicit maximum adaptation. (p. 785)
American Occupational Therapy Association. (1993). Position paper: Purposeful activity. *American Journal of Occupational Therapy, 47,* 1081–1082.	Occupation refers to active participation in self-maintenance, work, leisure, and play. Purposeful activity refers to goal-directed behaviors or tasks that comprise occupations. (p. 1081)
American Occupational Therapy Association. (1994). Uniform terminology for occupational therapy—third edition. *American Journal of Occupational Therapy, 48,* 1047–1054.	This document categorizes specific activities in each of the performance areas (ADL, work and productive activities, play or leisure). This categorization is based on what is considered "typical," and is not meant to imply that a particular individual characterizes personal activities in the same manner as someone else. Occupational therapy practitioners embrace individual differences, and so would document the unique pattern of the individual being served, rather than forcing the "typical" pattern on him or her and family. (p. 1048)
American Occupational Therapy Association. (1995). Concept paper: Service delivery in occupational therapy. *American Journal of Occupational Therapy, 49,* 1029–1031.	Since the time of occupational therapy's founding, the term *occupation* has been used to refer to an individual's active participation in self-maintenance, work, leisure, and play. . . . This paper's intent is to distinguish the term *occupation* from other terms, to summarize traditional beliefs about its nature and its therapeutic value, and to identify factors that have impeded the study and discussion of occupation. (p. 1015)
American Occupational Therapy Association. (1995). Position paper: Occupation. *American Journal of Occupational Therapy, 49,* 1015–1018.	Premises. 1) Service delivery is client-centered and recognizes the client's needs, wants, and priorities. 2) Service delivery involves the occupational therapy practitioner and client in a collaborative process of working together to design

(continues)

Table 1-1   Resources That Support Occupation-Based Practice. *(continued)*

DOCUMENT	QUOTATION
	and implement services. . . . 4) A client-centered perspective recognizes that the occupational therapy practitioner's interventions focus on performance in occupational activities (activities of daily living, work and productive activities, play or leisure activities) that meet the needs of the client. (p. 1029)
American Occupational Therapy Association. (1995). Position paper: Occupational performance: Occupational therapy's definition of function. *American Journal of Occupational Therapy, 49,* 1019–1020.	The concept of function and occupation remains at the core of occupational therapy. . . . (p. 1019) The unique contribution of occupational therapy is that the practitioner creates the opportunity for individuals to gain the skill and confidence to accomplish activities and tasks that are meaningful and productive, and in doing so, increases their occupational performance, thus their function. (p. 1020)
American Occupational Therapy Association. (1997). Fundamental concepts of occupational therapy: Occupation, purposeful activity, and function. *American Journal of Occupational Therapy, 51,* 864–866.	Occupational therapists use the term "occupation" to organize and define the profession's domain of concern. . . . Occupations are the activities people engage in throughout their daily lives to fulfill their time and give life meaning. . . . (p. 864) Occupational therapy practitioners need to keep the individual's occupations in the forefront of their thoughts when using any purposeful activity, and to plan interventions toward improving the individual's ability to function within his or her occupations. In the interest of the profession, it is important to concentrate on occupation. (p. 865)
American Occupational Therapy Association. (1998). Standards of practice for occupational therapy. *American Journal of Occupational Therapy, 52,* 866–869.	A registered occupational therapist [and a certified occupational therapy assistant under the supervision of a registered occupational therapist] implements the intervention plan through the use of specified purposeful activities or therapeutic methods that are meaningful to the client and are effective methods for enhancing occupational performance. (p. 868)
American Occupational Therapy Association. (2002). Occupational therapy practice framework: Domain and process. *American Journal of Occupational Therapy, 56,* 609–639.	Occupations are generally viewed as activities having unique meaning and purpose in a person's life. Occupations are central to a person's identity and competence, and they influence how one spends time and makes decisions. (p. 610) Engagement in occupation to support participation in context is the focus and targeted end objective of occupational therapy intervention. (p. 611)

occupation-based practice and includes excerpts relevant to occupation-based practice from each of the documents. The list is not intended to be all-inclusive. Resources are listed from earliest to most recent by publication date.

In addition to the resources within our profession, there are also supporting influences external to occupational therapy of which practitioners should be aware. The Balanced Budget Act (BBA) of 1997 has led to significant practice changes for practitioners in long-term care, outpatient, and home care practice settings. The changes not only reflect shifts in reimbursement, including prospective payment and capitation models, but also require skilled services to focus on the achievement of functional outcomes. Occupational therapy practitioners focus on the achievement of a client's functional outcomes through the use of meaningful and relevant occupations.

On an international level, the International Classification of Functioning, Disability and Health (ICF) (World Health Organization [WHO], 2001) focuses on an individual's performance and capacity, what an individual does in his or her current environment, and an individual's ability to execute a task or an action (WHO, 2001, p. 123). The ICF model recognizes that health can be affected by the inability to perform activities or occupations and participate in life situations. From an occupational therapy perspective the execution of occupations (functioning) by an individual or the difficulties an individual may have in executing occupations (disability) would fall under the functioning and disability section of the ICF model that consists of the life areas (tasks, actions) domain. This perspective parallels occupational therapy's focus on engagement in occupations to better an individual's occupational performance (AOTA, 2002) and can assist the practitioner in organizing service and documenting outcomes. "In fact, the unique feature of the profession is its belief that active participation in occupation is life itself" (Mandel, Jackson, Zemke, Nelson, & Clark, 1999, p. 12).

Summary

Putting occupation in your practice is often easier said than done. Educating and even reminding ourselves about the presence of occupation throughout the history and literature of the profession only begins the process. Focusing on, talking about, and understanding the influence that occupation has on health and well-being is essential. We need to talk about and demonstrate the power of occupation with everyone with whom we come into contact—our clients and their families, our colleagues—both occupational therapy practitioners and other health care professionals, our family members and friends, payers, legislators, and all members of our communities. As occupational therapy practitioners, we are the occupation experts and it is our responsibility to educate others about our expertise.

Occupation-based practice requires knowing what people do in their daily lives, what motivates people, and how personal characteristics combine with the life situations in which people execute occupations to influence performance (Baum, 2000). In the next chapter we will address the client-centered approach, which can assist the practitioner in gaining the unique information required to implement occupation-based practice.

References

American Occupational Therapy Association. (1979). The philosophical base of occupational therapy. *American Journal of Occupational Therapy, 33,* 785.

American Occupational Therapy Association. (1993). Position paper: Purposeful activity. *American Journal of Occupational Therapy, 47,* 1081–1082.

American Occupational Therapy Association. (1994). Uniform terminology for occupational therapy—third edition. *American Journal of Occupational Therapy, 48,* 1047–1054.

American Occupational Therapy Association. (1995). Concept paper: Service delivery in occupational therapy. *American Journal of Occupational Therapy, 49,* 1029–1031.

American Occupational Therapy Association. (1995). Position paper: Occupation. *American Journal of Occupational Therapy, 49,* 1015–1018.

American Occupational Therapy Association. (1995). Position paper: Occupational performance: Occupational therapy's definition of function. *American Journal of Occupational Therapy, 49,* 1019–1020.

American Occupational Therapy Association. (1997). Fundamental concepts of occupational therapy: Occupation, purposeful activity, and function. *American Journal of Occupational Therapy, 51,* 864–866.

American Occupational Therapy Association. (1998). Standards of practice for occupational therapy. *American Journal of Occupational Therapy, 52,* 866–869.

American Occupational Therapy Association. (2002). Occupational therapy practice framework: Domain and process. *American Journal of Occupational Therapy, 56,* 609–639.

Baum, C. (2000, January 3). Occupation-based practice: Reinventing ourselves for the new millennium. *OT Practice, 5*(1), 12–15.

Baum, C., & Baptiste, S. (2002). Reframing occupational therapy practice. In M. Law, C. M. Baum, & S. Baptiste, *Occupation-based practice: Fostering performance and participation* (pp. 3–15). Thorofare, NJ: Slack, Inc.

Clark, F., Parham, D., Carlson, M., Frank, G., Jackson, J., Pierce, D., et al. (1991). Occupational science: Academic innovation in the service of occupational therapy's future. *American Journal of Occupational Therapy, 45,* 300–310.

Law, M., Polatajko, H., Baptiste, S., & Townsend, E. (1997). Core concepts of occupational therapy. In E. Townsend (Ed.), *Enabling occupation: An occupational therapy perspective* (pp. 29–56). Ottawa, ON: CAOT Publishers, ACE.

Mandel, D. R., Jackson, J., Zemke, R., Nelson, L., & Clark, F. (1999). *Lifestyle redesign: Implementing the well elderly program.* Bethesda, MD: American Occupational Therapy Association, Inc.

Peloquin, S. M. (1991). Occupational therapy service: Individual and collective understandings of the founders, part 2. *American Journal of Occupational Therapy, 45,* 733–744.

World Health Organization. (2001). ICF: International classification of functioning, disability and health. Geneva: Author.

Suggested Readings

In addition to the references listed in this chapter, the following are useful information sources for occupation-based practice.

Crist, P. A., Royeen, C. B., & Schkade, J. K. (2000). *Infusing occupation into practice* (2nd ed.). Bethesda, MD: American Occupational Therapy Association, Inc.

Fazio, L. (2001). *Developing occupation-centered programs for the community: A workbook for students and professionals.* Upper Saddle River, NJ: Prentice-Hall, Inc.

Hasselkus, B. R. (2002). *The meaning of everyday occupation.* Thorofare, NJ: Slack, Inc.

Law, M., Baum, C. M., & Baptiste, S. (2002). *Occupation-based practice: Fostering performance and participation.* Thorofare, NJ: Slack, Inc.

Velde, B., & Fidler, G. (2002). *Lifestyle performance: A model for engaging in the power of occupation.* Thorofare, NJ: Slack, Inc.

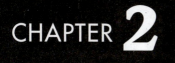

CHAPTER 2

A Client-Centered Approach

Learning Objectives

After reading this chapter and completing the learning activities, you should be able to do the following:

1. Define client-centered occupational therapy.
2. Identify strategies for implementing a client-centered approach in occupational therapy practice.
3. Describe a client-centered interview strategy.
4. Understand how the results of a client-centered interview influence the development of an occupation-based intervention plan.

Key Terms and Concepts

client-centered approach
client-centered interview

INTRODUCTION

The inclusion of a **client-centered approach** in occupation-based practice is essential. The client's experiences, values, priorities, and desired outcomes provide the structure for the inclusion of occupation-based interventions. This chapter provides an overview of client-centered practice, a client-centered interview strategy, an opportunity to trial the strategy, and a list of resources.

CLIENT-CENTERED PRACTICE

Client-centered practice has been defined as "an approach to service which embraces a philosophy of, respect for, and partnership with, people receiving services" (Law, Baptiste, & Mills, 1995, p. 253). Law and Mills (1998) identified concepts of client-centered practice common to all models of client-centered, patient-centered, and family-centered care. The concepts include the following:

➤ Respecting clients, as well as the choices they make.

➤ Understanding that clients have the ultimate responsibility for decisions about their daily occupations and services.

➤ Emphasizing person-centered communication.

➤ Facilitating client participation in service delivery.

➤ Delivering service that is flexible and individualized.

➤ Encouraging and empowering clients to solve occupational performance issues.

➤ Focusing on the relationship between the person, his or her environment, and his or her occupations.

These concepts, when incorporated into occupational therapy, form the foundation for occupation-based practice. A client-centered approach establishes a collaborative partnership between the practitioner and client. Typically a client seeks out or is referred to occupational therapy services when experiencing an occupational performance problem (i.e., difficulty performing or engaging in the occupations that support participation in his or her context[s]). It is important to note that the concept of the client is not restricted to the individual experiencing the occupational performance problem. The client may and often does include other individuals involved in supporting or caring for the individual with the occupational performance problem. The client-centered approach in occupation-based practice enables the practitioner to tailor the intervention plan to the experiences, values, priorities, and desired outcomes of the client.

Client-centered care is neither unique to occupational therapy nor health care. Perhaps without realizing it, you receive client-centered services as you perform your daily occupations. For example, when you go to the store to purchase a computer the first question the retail professional, whom we shall call Mike, typically asks is, "How can I help you?" Mike is engaging you in the collaborative relationship. You respond, "I would like to purchase a computer." Mike now gathers important and unique information from you in order to determine how he can best assist you in reaching your desired outcome of purchasing a computer. Mike asks probing questions such as "What tasks will you need to do with the computer?" and "What tasks do you want to do on the computer?" and "What tasks will you be expected to do using the computer?" These are relevant questions that help Mike to better understand your specific needs, wants, and expectations so that he is able to recommend appropriate computer products. Your responses to the three questions may overlap, however, a need is often different from a want, and both a need and a want often differ from an expectation. For example, you may want and need to have a software program on the computer that will enable you to make greeting cards. In addition, you may need to have a computer set-up that prevents physical strain because you are expected to work on your computer for extended periods of time. Or you may have responded that you want a computer that has fast processing capabilities, need a computer that is a specific size to fit your desk and is less than a specific cost, and are expected to have the computer up and running within a week.

Your responses enable Mike to identify computers that might address what you need to do, want to do, and/or are expected to do. But what if your responses to Mike's questions do not match the products that Mike has to offer? There may not be a "single" computer that meets all of your needs, wants, and expectations. In this case, Mike may have you prioritize what is most important to you in order to recommend the most appropriate or "best" computer to meet your needs, wants, and expectations. The end result is that you not only have purchased a computer (your desired outcome) but that you have purchased a computer that you are satisfied with and one that you are more motivated to use since it matches your needs, wants, and expectations.

A client-centered approach significantly enhances your ability as an occupational therapy practitioner to provide occupation-based intervention. Pollack and McColl (1998) identified a variety of assessment methods (i.e., informal interviews, narrative and life history, metaphor, semi-structured interview, and health and functional status questionnaires) that practitioners can use to identify occupational performance problems. The *Canadian Occupational Performance Measure* (COPM) (Law, et al., 1998) is an individualized outcome instrument designed to measure change in a client's self-perception of occupational performance over time. The COPM is a semi-structured interview tool that can assist practitioners in providing client-centered occupation-based intervention by helping them to identify and prioritize the occupations that a client needs to do, wants to do, and is expected to do. We support the use of the COPM in its entirety; however, if the inclusion of an additional tool is not desired or practical, we encourage practitioners to use the concepts established in the COPM during the assessment of a client's occupational performance problems. You can use the concepts in the COPM to assist you in incorporating a client-centered approach into your occupational therapy practice.

CLIENT-CENTERED INTERVIEW

The **client-centered interview** provides a strategy for obtaining information about your client's needs, wants, and expectations related to his or her occupational performance. This strategy can assist you in developing an occupation-based intervention plan for your client. The interview is conducted utilizing theoretical and practical effective communication and interview skills typically used in occupational therapy practice—such as preparation of the client and setting, attending and nurturing actions, listening and observation skills, appropriate use of social chitchat, paraphrasing, and use of questions and feedback (Denton, 1987). The practitioner is encouraged to develop an effective interviewing style that is comfortable for both the practitioner and client that elicits information about occupational performance issues. The following list outlines the steps of the client-centered interview process.

STEP 1:   Ask your client to think about the occupations he or she performs during a typical day and provide three to five responses to the following:

Occupations I need to do:

1.
2.
3.
4.
5.

Occupations I want to do:

1.
2.
3.
4.
5.

Occupations I am expected to do:

1.

2.

3.

4.

5.

STEP 2: Ask your client to circle his or her five most important occupations.

Prior to conducting the client-centered interview the practitioner must ensure that the client understands the definition of occupation from an occupational therapy perspective. Recall the definition of occupation from Chapter 1—"Occupations are generally viewed as activities having unique meaning and purpose in a person's life. Occupations are central to a person's identity and competence, and they influence how one spends time and makes decisions" (American Occupational Therapy Association, 2002). When explaining the concept of occupation to a client, use examples of occupations that are relevant to the client and span more than one area of occupation (i.e., activities of daily living, instrumental activities of daily living, education, work, play, leisure, and social participation). Ask clients to describe what they do during a typical day and use examples of their occupations to assist in defining and clarifying the concept of occupation. Refer to Appendix A for a list of areas of occupation.

Check Your Thinking 2-1

In order to better understand the utility of the client-centered interview strategy, you now have the opportunity to complete your own client-centered interview. Completing this learning exercise from *your* personal perspective will provide you with insight on how the client-centered interview is viewed from the client's perspective.

STEP 1: Think about the occupations you perform during a typical day and provide three to five responses to the following:

Occupations I need to do:

1.

2.

3.

4.

5.

Occupations I want to do:

1.

2.

3.

4.

5.

Occupations I am expected to do:

1.

2.

3.

4.

5.

STEP 2: Circle your five most important occupations.

Was it easy or difficult to identify your needs, wants, and expectations? Were there enough spaces under each area? Was it difficult to prioritize the occupations that are most important? Did you list the same or similar occupations under more than one category (i.e., needs, wants, and expectations)? Consider how your experience completing the client-centered interview may be similar to a client's experience. How might a client's experience differ from yours?

What Ifs

1. What if you fractured your wrist? Brainstorm a list of interventions that you might include in the occupational therapy intervention plan of a client with a diagnosis of a wrist fracture.

Refer to the results of your client-centered interview, which includes a list of the occupations you identified as needing, wanting, and being expected to perform and occupations you identified as priority areas. If you fractured the wrist of your dominant hand:

a. Which of your identified occupations would be affected?

b. Would your list of priority occupations change?

c. Would your list of interventions facilitate your ability to perform your prioritized occupations?

2. What if you had major depression? Brainstorm a list of interventions that you might include in the occupational therapy intervention plan of a client with a diagnosis of major depression.

Refer to the results of *your* client-centered interview, which includes a list of the occupations you identified as needing, wanting, and being expected to perform and occupations you identified as priority areas. If you had major depression:

a. Which of your identified occupations would be affected?

b. Would your list of priority occupations change?

c. Would your list of interventions facilitate your ability to perform your prioritized occupations?

Having reviewed and completed the learning exercises illustrating the client-centered interview strategy, you have started to build your occupation-based practice skills. It is important to remember that the focus of the client-centered approach is the *client*, not the practitioner. Occupational therapy practitioners must be able to retrieve relevant information from a client in order to plan and implement interventions that will assist in improving the client's occupational performance or engagement in occupations for participation in his or her context(s). Using client-centered tools and strategies, such as the COPM (Law et al., 1998) and a client-centered interview strategy, in your daily practice can assist you in obtaining the unique information necessary for developing an occupation-based intervention plan for each of your clients.

Summary

The results of the client-centered interview drive the development of the occupational therapy intervention plan. The intervention plan should support the occupations identified and prioritized by the client. Chapter 3 addresses the development of the intervention plan through use of the intervention continuum, and Chapter 7 provides you with the opportunity to practice developing occupational therapy intervention plans based on sample client-centered interviews in clinical scenarios that reflect a variety of clients and practice settings.

References

American Occupational Therapy Association. (2002). Occupational therapy practice framework: Domain and process. *American Journal of Occupational Therapy, 56,* 609–639.

Denton, P. L. (1987). Effective communication. In *Psychiatric occupational therapy: A workbook of practical skills* (pp. 1–40). Boston: Little, Brown and Company.

Law, M., Baptiste, S., Carswell, A., McColl, M. A., Polatajko, H., & Pollack, N. (1998). *Canadian Occupational Performance Measure* (3rd ed.). Ottawa, Ontario: CAOT Publications ACE.

Law, M., Baptiste, S., & Mills, J. (1995). Client-centered practice: What does it mean and does it make a difference? *Canadian Journal of Occupational Therapy, 62,* 250–257.

Law, M., & Mills, J. (1998). Client-centered occupational therapy. In M. Law (Ed.), *Client-centered occupational therapy* (pp. 1–18). Thorofare, NJ: Slack, Inc.

Pollack, N., & McColl, M. A. (1998). Assessment in client-centered occupational therapy. In M. Law (Ed.), *Client-centered occupational therapy* (pp. 89–105). Thorofare, NJ: Slack, Inc.

Suggested Readings

In addition to the references listed in this chapter, the following are useful information sources for client-centered practice.

Fearing, V. G., & Clark. J. (Eds.). (2000). *Individuals in context: A practical guide to client-centered practice.* Thorofare, NJ: Slack, Inc.

Sumsion, T. (1999). *Client-centred practice in occupational therapy: A guide to implementation.* Philadelphia: Churchill Livingstone.

CHAPTER 3

The Intervention Continuum

Learning Objectives

After reading this chapter and completing the learning activities, you should be able to do the following:

1. Describe the categories of the intervention continuum (adjunctive interventions, enabling interventions, purposeful interventions, and occupation-based interventions).
2. Identify and categorize interventions as being adjunctive, enabling, purposeful, and/or occupation-based.
3. Describe how the same interventions may be categorized differently for different clients.
4. Describe how the intervention continuum can be used as a clinical reasoning tool for choosing appropriate client-centered interventions.

Key Terms and Concepts

intervention continuum
adjunctive interventions
enabling interventions
purposeful interventions
occupation-based interventions

INTRODUCTION

Information gathered during the occupational therapy evaluation process guides intervention planning and the identification of outcome-oriented goals. This information directs occupational therapy practitioners in the selection of appropriate interventions. As such, client-centered intervention planning is a requisite of occupation-based practice and supports one of the profession's basic tenets, the use of occupation as a means toward recovery and wellness. This chapter describes an **intervention continuum** that occupational therapy practitioners can use to categorize interventions to determine if the occupational therapy intervention plan is directed toward engaging the client in occupations to support participation. The examples of interventions provided in this chapter are not intended to reflect best practice nor are they meant to be all-inclusive. They are designed to provide guidance for the categorization of interventions.

CLASSIFICATION IN THE INTERVENTION CONTINUUM

Pedretti (1996a) described a treatment continuum for adults with physical disabilities based on the Occupational Performance Model. Pedretti's treatment continuum includes a description of adjunctive, enabling, purposeful, and occupation-based activities. The intervention continuum (Chisholm, Dolhi, & Schreiber, 2000b) discussed in this manual uses Pedretti's model as a foundation and expands the continuum to include a wide range of age and diagnostic considerations across occupational therapy practice settings.

CLINICAL SCENARIO—BEN

The following clinical scenario is used to illustrate the intervention continuum and will be referred to in the discussion of each category.

Occupational Profile and Analysis of Occupational Performance

Ben is a 38-year-old, right-hand dominant, biology teacher who sustained a closed head injury after falling from a rooftop. Ben lives with his wife and 3-year-old son in a two-story home with an attached garage. Prior to his injury, Ben was independent with all self-care tasks and actively participated in caring for his son. He was responsible for the yard work and automotive care and assisted his wife with the indoor home management tasks. Ben worked for his brother's contracting company during the summer months. He drove and routinely accompanied his wife on shopping trips. He was involved in a weekly men's basketball league, played golf occasionally, and enjoyed stock car racing. Ben was referred to occupational therapy upon his admission to the rehabilitation center. Ben presents with left side hemiparesis. His left upper extremity strength is fair + at the shoulder and fair for elbow flexion/extension and wrist flexion/extension. He is unable to complete fist closure or maintain grasp. He also exhibits edema in the left hand. Left lower extremity strength is fair for all major muscle groups. Ben's strength and range of motion of the right extremities are within normal limits. His vision and perception are intact. Mild impairments are noted in short-term memory and problem-solving skills. Ben performs toilet, chair, and bed transfers with minimal assistance. He is able to complete grooming and feeding after set-up. Ben needs minimal assistance to pull a shirt over his head and down his back. He performs lower extremity dressing with moderate assistance secondary to requiring set-up for retrieval of items, decreased standing balance, and left side weakness. Ben ambulates with a quad cane and moderate assistance. After a brief discussion regarding Ben's social history, roles, and occupations, he participated in a client-centered interview.

Ben's Client-Centered Interview Results

The following is Ben's client-centered interview, which includes a list of the occupations that he identified as needing, wanting, and being expected to perform. The occupations Ben identified as priority areas for improvement are circled.

Occupations I need to do:

(1.) Return to teaching

2. Bathe and dress myself

(3.) Drive

4. Help my wife with household chores

(5.) Take care of my son

Occupations I want to do:

(1.) Make lunch for my son

2. Play basketball

3. Play golf

4. Take my son to the park and push him on a swing

5. Drive my car

Occupations I am expected to do:

1. Take care of my son (including dressing, bathing, lunch preparation, play activities)

2. Take care of our lawn

3. Take care of our cars

4. Work as a biology teacher

(5.) Take care of myself (toileting, bathing, feeding, dressing, etc.)

ADJUNCTIVE INTERVENTION

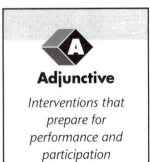

Adjunctive

Interventions that prepare for performance and participation

Adjunctive interventions represent the first phase of the intervention continuum. They are typically used to prepare a client for participation in a purposeful or an occupation-based intervention (American Occupational Therapy Association, 1997). Adjunctive interventions have been used successfully to address skill impairments such as strength, endurance, and range of motion (Bajuk, Jelnikar, & Ortar, 1996; Maddy & Meyerdierks, 1997).

Consider the clinical scenario of Ben. The occupational therapy practitioner may use a contrast bath in an attempt to decrease edema in Ben's left hand at the start of the therapy session. The contrast bath can be an appropriate intervention to include at this point in Ben's occupational therapy intervention plan. However, the contrast bath (or other adjunctive interventions) should not be the main focus or only category of intervention included in Ben's occupational therapy program. The unique contribution of occupational therapy is the use of occupation. Adjunctive interventions alone do not fulfill this unique role. Occupational therapy practitioners should use adjunctive interventions with the goal of preparing the client for participation in his or her occupations as identified during the client-centered interview.

The following are examples of adjunctive interventions:

➤ Massage

➤ Contrast bath

➤ Facilitation techniques (i.e., vibration and tapping)

➤ Orthotic devices

➤ Neurodevelopmental handling techniques

➤ Education—the presentation of written and/or verbal information

➤ Adaptive equipment—issuing or viewing

➤ Passive stretch

➤ Sensory integrative techniques (i.e., swinging, spinning, and deep pressure)

➤ Fluidotherapy

Helpful Hint: *Adjunctive = A is at the beginning* Adjunctive interventions are at the beginning of the intervention continuum and are typically used before engaging the client in other categories of interventions. "A" is at the beginning of the alphabet and before all of the other letters.

Check Your Thinking 3-1

Make a list of other adjunctive interventions.

Check Your Thinking 3-2

Adjunctive

Interventions that prepare for performance and participation

Identify the interventions that may be categorized as adjunctive by writing an A on the appropriate line. The answers can be found in Appendix B.

_____	dowel rod exercises
_____	scar massage
_____	pulling small pegs out of putty
_____	hot or ice pack
_____	placing pegs in a peg board
_____	issuing a handout listing stress management strategies
_____	paraffin wax dips
_____	upper extremity exercises with a resistive band
_____	compression wrap to decrease edema
_____	baking cookies in the occupational therapy kitchen
_____	handwriting exercises
_____	providing a letter strip for student's desk
_____	stacking cones
_____	bean bag toss game
_____	issuing adaptive equipment
_____	loading dishes in the occupational therapy department dishwasher
_____	fabricating and fitting a splint
_____	providing teachers with information related to sensory integration techniques
_____	wheelchair positioning techniques
_____	shoulder range of motion arc
_____	written information for caregivers
_____	discussion of relaxation techniques and brainstorming of potential applications
_____	locating and removing items from a rice bin
_____	stringing beads to make a necklace
_____	finger ladder
_____	styling hair with own supplies
_____	folding towels that belong to the occupational therapy clinic
_____	copying a paragraph from a magazine
_____	safety obstacle course
_____	cleaning the mirror in the occupational therapy bathroom

Check Your Thinking 3-3

Based on Ben's occupational profile and analysis of occupational performance, and his client-centered interview results, identify an area of occupation (refer to Appendix A) that is a priority for Ben. What adjunctive interventions could you include in Ben's occupational therapy intervention plan to prepare him for participation in the occupation you identified?

Area of occupation:

Adjunctive interventions:

ENABLING INTERVENTION

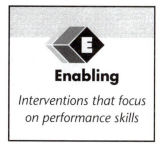

Enabling

Interventions that focus on performance skills

Enabling interventions refer to those interventions used in a therapy session that would appear to simulate an activity and are not directly purposeful, but incorporate the use and integration of performance skills (Pedretti & Early, 2001). Enabling interventions are similar to adjunctive interventions in that they are used to remediate skill impairments in order to enhance a client's active participation in occupations. An enabling intervention focuses on the performance of select skills, whereas an adjunctive intervention is used to prepare the client for skill performance.

An example of an enabling intervention frequently used by occupational therapy practitioners is upper extremity exercise. For example, Ben may perform exercises in order to increase range of motion and strength in his left arm. The exercise program may be designed to strengthen the motions required for meal preparation, such as opening food containers and kitchen cabinets, or lifting and transporting food and cooking utensils. The exercises may assist Ben in improving his skill performance in order to achieve an occupation he identified as a priority during his client-centered interview ("prepare lunch for my son").

When the occupational therapy practitioner includes enabling (and/or adjunctive) interventions that support the performance of the client's occupations, the practitioner has the opportunity to emphasize the importance of occupation with the client both verbally and in performance. Explaining to Ben that the muscles and movements involved in meal preparation are the same muscles and movements incorporated in the arm exercises can be motivating and emphasizes the meaning and relevance of occupational therapy services in facilitating his health and participation in desired occupations.

Exercise can be an appropriate enabling intervention to include in Ben's intervention plan. However, exercises or enabling interventions should not be the main focus or the only interventions included in Ben's occupational therapy program. Remember, the unique contribution of occupational therapy is the use of occupation. As with adjunctive interventions, enabling interventions alone do not fulfill this unique role. Occupational therapy practitioners should use enabling interventions with the goal of preparing the client for participation in his or her occupations as identified during the client-centered interview.

The following are examples of enabling interventions:

➤ Circling letters on a scanning sheet
➤ Graded Pinch Exercises
➤ Dressing board
➤ Hand warm-ups for writing
➤ Completing cognitive worksheet activities
➤ Verbal instruction with demonstration
➤ Range of motion or strengthening exercises
➤ Practicing the operation of adaptive equipment
➤ Replicating parquetry block designs
➤ Using therapy putty to increase hand strength

> **Helpful Hint:** *Enabling = exercise-oriented* Enabling interventions can be used to improve those skill deficits that may be remediated through exercise-oriented interventions. Enabling begins with "E," as does exercise-oriented. Remember that different types of exercises can be used to address a variety of skill impairments (e.g., sensorimotor, neuromusculoskeletal, motor, cognition, psychosocial/ psychological).

Check Your Thinking 3-4

Make a list of other enabling interventions.

Check Your Thinking 3-5

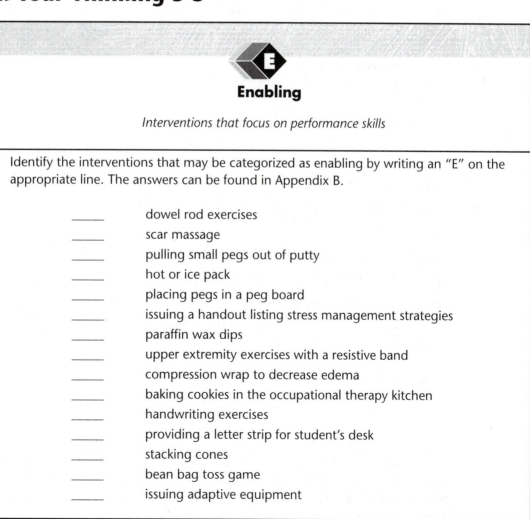

Enabling

Interventions that focus on performance skills

Identify the interventions that may be categorized as enabling by writing an "E" on the appropriate line. The answers can be found in Appendix B.

_____	dowel rod exercises
_____	scar massage
_____	pulling small pegs out of putty
_____	hot or ice pack
_____	placing pegs in a peg board
_____	issuing a handout listing stress management strategies
_____	paraffin wax dips
_____	upper extremity exercises with a resistive band
_____	compression wrap to decrease edema
_____	baking cookies in the occupational therapy kitchen
_____	handwriting exercises
_____	providing a letter strip for student's desk
_____	stacking cones
_____	bean bag toss game
_____	issuing adaptive equipment

(continues)

(continued)

Enabling

_____	loading dishes in the occupational therapy department dishwasher
_____	fabricating and fitting a splint
_____	providing teachers with information related to sensory integration techniques
_____	wheelchair positioning techniques
_____	shoulder range of motion arc
_____	written information for caregivers
_____	discussion of relaxation techniques and brainstorming of potential applications
_____	locating and removing items from a rice bin
_____	stringing beads to make a necklace
_____	finger ladder
_____	styling hair with own supplies
_____	folding towels that belong to the occupational therapy clinic
_____	copying a paragraph from a magazine
_____	safety obstacle course
_____	cleaning the mirror in the occupational therapy bathroom

Check Your Thinking 3-6

Based on Ben's occupational profile and analysis of occupational performance, and his client-centered interview results, identify an area of occupation (refer to Appendix A) that is a priority for Ben. What enabling interventions could you include in Ben's occupational therapy intervention plan to address performance skill impairments required for participation in the occupation you identified?

Area of occupation:

Enabling interventions:

PURPOSEFUL INTERVENTION

Purposeful

Interventions that have a pre-determined goal and facilitate practice and problem solving

The "Philosophical Base of Occupational Therapy" (American Occupational Therapy Association, 1979) includes the integration of **purposeful interventions** in therapy. The use of purposeful activities or interventions has historically served to distinguish occupational therapy from other health care professions (Ayres, 1958).

A purposeful intervention is an intervention that has a predetermined goal and an obvious beginning and end. Like adjunctive and enabling interventions, purposeful interventions can be used to remediate skill impairments. However, unlike adjunctive and enabling interventions, purposeful interventions focus on the improvement of areas of occupation (American Occupational Therapy Association, 1993; Pedretti, 1996b; Pedretti & Early, 2001). Occupational therapy practitioners often use purposeful interventions following adjunctive and/or enabling interventions. For example, because Ben presented with increased edema in his left hand, the occupational therapy practitioner provided a contrast bath (adjunctive intervention) in order to decrease the swelling. Next, Ben performed active range of motion exercises (enabling intervention). Although Ben's occupational therapy practitioner appropriately included adjunctive and enabling interventions that are useful for improving skill impairments (e.g., range of motion and gross grasp) in his intervention program, the need remains for Ben to integrate his improved skills in order to perform his occupations.

Purposeful interventions can be used to assist Ben in integrating skill performance. After performing arm exercises (enabling intervention), Ben's therapy may include removing various sized and shaped lids from empty food containers. This purposeful intervention can facilitate integration of multiple skills (e.g., sensorimotor, neuromusculoskeletal, motor, cognition, and psychosocial/psychological). This intervention is purposeful as it has a predetermined goal (remove lids from empty food containers), a beginning (start with lids secured on empty food containers), and an obvious end (task is completed when the lids are removed from empty food containers). Opening empty food containers can be an appropriate purposeful intervention to include in Ben's occupational therapy services as it promotes the performance of one of his desired occupations—preparing lunch for his son. As with all purposeful interventions, opening empty food containers challenges a range of performance skills. In contrast to the adjunctive intervention (contrast bath) and enabling intervention (upper extremity exercises) included in Ben's therapy session, the purposeful intervention (opening empty food containers) directly addresses an area of occupation (meal preparation). So far Ben has performed interventions in three categories (i.e., adjunctive, enabling, and purposeful) of the intervention continuum.

The following are examples of purposeful interventions:

➤ Making a sandwich in the clinic kitchen
➤ Practicing dressing using facility clothes
➤ Wiping clinic tables
➤ Scooter board obstacle course
➤ Playing adapted checkers with therapist
➤ Crafts
➤ Copying a paragraph from a magazine
➤ Role-playing anger management strategies
➤ Simulated money transactions
➤ Gift wrapping an empty box

> **Helpful Hint:** *Purposeful = practice and problem solving* Purposeful interventions have a goal, a beginning, and an end, and their purpose is to facilitate the client's practice and problem solving of his or her occupations. However, purposeful interventions do not necessarily reflect the client's priority occupations nor the client's typical performance contexts.

Check Your Thinking 3-7

Make a list of other purposeful interventions.

Check Your Thinking 3-8

Purposeful

Interventions that have a pre-determined goal and facilitate practice and problem solving

Identify the interventions that may be categorized as purposeful by writing a "P" on the appropriate line. The answers can be found in Appendix B.

_____	dowel rod exercises
_____	scar massage
_____	pulling small pegs out of putty
_____	hot or ice pack
_____	placing pegs in a peg board
_____	issuing a handout listing stress management strategies
_____	paraffin wax dips
_____	upper extremity exercises with a resistive band
_____	compression wrap to decrease edema
_____	baking cookies in the occupational therapy kitchen
_____	handwriting exercises

(continues)

(continued)

Purposeful

_____ providing a letter strip for student's desk

_____ stacking cones

_____ bean bag toss game

_____ issuing adaptive equipment

_____ loading dishes in the occupational therapy department dishwasher

_____ fabricating and fitting a splint

_____ providing teachers with information related to sensory integration techniques

_____ wheelchair positioning techniques

_____ shoulder range of motion arc

_____ written information for caregivers

_____ discussion of relaxation techniques and brainstorming of potential applications

_____ locating and removing items from a rice bin

_____ stringing beads to make a necklace

_____ finger ladder

_____ styling hair with own supplies

_____ folding towels that belong to the occupational therapy clinic

_____ copying a paragraph from a magazine

_____ safety obstacle course

_____ cleaning the mirror in the occupational therapy bathroom

Check Your Thinking 3-9

Based on Ben's occupational profile and analysis of occupational performance, and his client-centered interview results, identify an area of occupation (refer to Appendix A) that is a priority for Ben. What purposeful interventions could you include in Ben's occupational therapy intervention plan that would allow him the opportunity to practice and problem solve steps of the occupation you identified?

Area of occupation:

```



```

Purposeful interventions:

OCCUPATION-BASED INTERVENTION

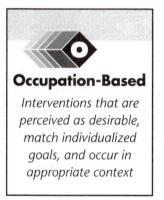

Occupation-Based

Interventions that are perceived as desirable, match individualized goals, and occur in appropriate context

Occupational therapy is a health care profession that focuses on how people occupy their time, that is, the occupations they perform. Occupational therapy practitioners use occupations as a means to remediate and/or compensate for activity limitations and/or participation restrictions. Occupational therapy is ideally discontinued when the client has achieved the maximal level of performance of his or her daily occupations within the appropriate contexts or environments. By evaluating the client's ability to perform and participate in his or her occupations, the occupational therapy practitioner creates an intervention plan that includes therapeutic methods not only effective for facilitating maximal occupational performance in life roles, but those that are meaningful to the client.

As stated earlier in this manual, establishing and providing **occupation-based interventions** can present a challenge for practitioners at all levels of experience. The inclusion of occupation-based interventions in a client's occupational therapy intervention plan requires a clear and accurate understanding of the occupations the client perceives as needing to, wanting to, and being expected to perform (Chisholm, Dolhi, & Schreiber, 2000a; Law et al., 1998). Although a challenge, the use of occupation-based intervention is recognized as being the most beneficial for the generalization of occupations (Clark et al., 1997; Kleinman & Stalcup, 1991). An occupation-based intervention is defined as an intervention that is perceived by the client as desirable, matching his or her personal goals, and occurring in its appropriate context (Pierce, 1998). It may be difficult to achieve all of these elements in some practice settings. The occupational therapy practitioner is encouraged to address as many of the elements as possible when designing the client's occupational therapy intervention plan. Occupation-based interventions may be used at any and all points in the client's occupational therapy intervention plan. Incorporation of occupation-based interventions may be used to meet outcome-related short-term goals or to attain the skills necessary to reach a separate long-term goal (Gray, 1998).

At this point you might be thinking, how do I differentiate between a purposeful intervention and an occupation-based intervention? These interventions seem like they could be categorized the same. It can be difficult to distinguish between the purposeful and occupation-based categories for a particular intervention. An intervention that appears to be purposeful may actually be occupation-based and vice versa, depending on the specifics of the client and clinical situation. The following scenario should help to clarify this issue.

Recall our client Ben. Both Ben and another client, Sarah, identified meal preparation as a priority occupation in their client-centered interviews. Therefore, both Ben's and Sarah's occupational therapy intervention plans include goals related to meal preparation. The occupational therapy practitioner includes preparing boxed macaroni and cheese in one of their therapy sessions. Most practitioners would agree that this intervention could be appropriately used to address the occupation of meal preparation and a variety of performance skill impairments (e.g., postural control, memory, gross and fine coordination, problem solving, safety, endurance, and role performance).

Sarah performs the meal preparation intervention although she dislikes macaroni and cheese and has no intention of eating the meal or preparing it in the future. This intervention is a purposeful intervention for Sarah—the intervention has a goal, a beginning, and an end, and addresses multiple performance skills as well as an area of occupation. However, it does not fall into the occupation-based intervention category for her because it has no personal meaning to Sarah, who dislikes macaroni and cheese and has no intention of eating the meal or preparing it in the future. When the occupational therapy practitioner includes a purposeful intervention that supports the performance of Sarah's (or any client's) occupations, the practitioner again has the opportunity to emphasize the importance of occupation both verbally and in performance. Explain to Sarah that performance skills needed to prepare her favorite meal of vegetable lasagna are the same skills she is using when preparing macaroni and cheese. Understanding the relationship between performance of an intervention and her occupations can be motivating and emphasizes the meaning and relevance of occupational therapy services in facilitating her health and participation in her desired occupations.

Ben, however, likes macaroni and cheese and also regularly prepares it for his son. For Ben, this meal preparation intervention is categorized as an occupation-based intervention because the task of preparing boxed macaroni and cheese has personal meaning for him, that is, he not only likes it but he also regularly prepares it for his son. Remember the elements of occupation-based intervention include being perceived by the client as desirable, matching the client's personal goals, and occurring in its appropriate context (Pierce, 1998). For Ben, preparing macaroni and cheese is desirable and matches at least one of his personal goals or priority occupations (preparing lunch for his son). Although the appropriate context for Ben to prepare macaroni and cheese would be his kitchen, using his utensils and appliances, the occupational therapy practitioner is striving to achieve the highest level of occupation-based intervention possible within the environmental constraints of the clinic setting (i.e., only having access to the clinic kitchen and clinic utensils and appliances).

Our client, Ben, has participated in interventions across the intervention continuum—contrast bath (adjunctive intervention), exercise (enabling intervention), opening food containers (purposeful intervention), and preparation of macaroni and cheese (occupation-based intervention). In order for occupation-based interventions to facilitate Ben's optimal performance in his desired occupation, the practitioner must consider the following: environment (context), objects (materials), and time. The practitioner should attempt to match as close as possible the natural environment in which the client performs the occupation, the objects the client uses to perform the occupation, and the time when the client typically performs the occupation. Table 3-1 compares the context, materials, and time factors of an occupation-based intervention and an occupation. In Ben's situation, the macaroni and cheese intervention would be his occupation if it were conducted in his kitchen, with his own kitchen tools, and during the usual time he prepares and consumes his meal. However, the occupational therapy practitioner has facilitated the use of occupation-based intervention at the highest level based on the constraints of the practice setting—Ben's kitchen and kitchen tools are not available in the clinic nor can therapy sessions always be scheduled during mealtime. Additionally, if the occupational therapy practitioner discusses with Ben elements of how he prepares macaroni and cheese in his home environment and facilitates problem solving of potential barriers he might encounter when performing meal preparation, the practitioner has maximized the occupation-based intervention in order to support Ben's ability to perform his desired occupation—meal preparation.

When practice is occupation-based, a plan is developed that includes interventions designed to promote the performance of the client's desired occupations. The occupational therapy plan may appropriately include interventions from all of the

Table 3-1	Comparing Context, Materials, and Time of an Occupation-Based Intervention and an Occupation.	
	BEN'S OCCUPATION-BASED INTERVENTION	**BEN'S OCCUPATION**
Context	Unfamiliar clinic kitchen	Ben's kitchen
Materials	Unfamiliar cooking pans and utensils	Ben's cooking pans and utensils
Time	Performed during scheduled therapy session; not meal time	Performed at Ben's typical meal preparation time

categories in the intervention continuum. However, the objective should not necessarily be to involve the client in each intervention type, but to include interventions that facilitate the client's highest level of engagement in occupation to support participation in context(s).

The following are examples of occupation-based interventions:

➤ Laundering own clothes
➤ Copying a desired recipe from a magazine
➤ Telephoning a friend
➤ Typing own resume
➤ Sewing a button on own shirt
➤ Purchasing desired items from the gift shop
➤ Transferring from own wheelchair to own car
➤ Playing checkers with a family member
➤ Cleaning sink area after performing morning grooming tasks
➤ Socializing with peers during age-appropriate activities

> **Helpful Hint:** *Occupation-based = ownership* Occupation-based interventions address those occupations that are personally meaningful to the client. Therefore, the client takes ownership of his or her occupations.

Check Your Thinking 3-10

Make a list of other occupation-based interventions.

Check Your Thinking 3-11

Ben identified the following as priority occupations for improvement after sustaining a closed head injury:

✔ Return to teaching

✔ Drive

✔ Take care of my son

✔ Make lunch for my son

✔ Take care of myself (toileting, bathing, feeding, dressing, etc.)

Occupation-Based

Interventions that are perceived as desirable, match individualized goals, and occur in appropriate context

Identify the interventions that may be categorized as occupation-based for Ben by writing an "O" on the appropriate line. The answers can be found in Appendix B.

_____	lifting a crate that weighs as much as his child
_____	completing grooming while standing at the sink
_____	making dinner for his wife
_____	placing pegs in a peg board
_____	completing upper extremity exercise for affected arm
_____	transcribing class notes on a chalkboard
_____	transferring in and out of own car in facility parking lot
_____	folding towels that belong to the occupational therapy department
_____	contrast bath
_____	copying a recipe for beef although he dislikes meat
_____	dribbling a basketball on the facility basketball court
_____	preparing his child's favorite lunch meal
_____	preparing notes from biology book
_____	pulling small pegs out of putty
_____	standing in a standing box to increase standing endurance

Check Your Thinking 3-12

Based on Ben's occupational profile and analysis of occupational performance, and his client-centered interview results, identify an area of occupation (refer to Appendix A) that is a priority for Ben. What occupation-based interventions could you include in Ben's occupational therapy intervention plan that would be desirable to him, match his personal goals, and/or occur in the appropriate context of his occupation?

Area of occupation:

Occupation-based interventions:

Summary

Becoming an occupation-based practitioner takes practice. Planning and implementing occupational therapy intervention plans that include occupation-based interventions may initially require more time and thought; however, with practice, the inclusion of occupation-based interventions can become the standard in your clinical habit pattern. Chapter 7 will give you the opportunity to practice planning client-centered occupational therapy plans using the intervention continuum as a tool for clinical reasoning.

As you begin to put the pieces together—occupations, a client-centered approach, the intervention continuum, and occupation-based interventions—through completion of the clinical scenario exercises in Chapter 7 and in the planning and implementation of the "real-life" clients of your clinical practice, consider the following:

➤ Although the categories of the intervention continuum have been presented sequentially (i.e., adjunctive intervention followed by enabling intervention, then purposeful intervention, and finally occupation-based intervention), it is not required that interventions be provided in this sequence. It may be appropriate for the occupational therapy practitioner to omit or return to intervention categories during the therapy program with a specific client. The sequence of the continuum is only a guide for facilitating the inclusion of occupation-based interventions.

➤ It may not be appropriate or realistic to address each of the four categories of the intervention continuum within one intervention session or the therapy program.

➤ The same intervention may be categorized differently for different clients, especially within the purposeful and occupation-based intervention categories. Categorization of an intervention is dependent on the client's occupational profile and analysis of occupational performance, and the client's occupations (i.e., the daily activities that the client perceives as needing, wanting, and being expected to perform).

➤ Interventions in the adjunctive or enabling categories of the continuum may be beneficial in the remediation of performance skill impairments (e.g., sensorimotor, neuromusculoskeletal, motor, cognition, psychosocial/psychological) but do not inherently promote generalization toward performance of the client's occupations (e.g., dressing, meal preparation and clean-up, care of pets, job performance, and family and peer interactions). Occupational therapy practitioners should use adjunctive and enabling interventions as precursors to engaging the client in purposeful and occupation-based interventions.

➤ Occupation-based intervention is not limited to basic activities of daily living (i.e., dressing, bathing, and grooming). Occupational therapy practitioners are urged to broaden their scope of interventions to cover the range of occupations (i.e., activities of daily living, instrumental activities of daily living, education, work, play, leisure, and social participation) appropriate for the specific client.

➤ Occupational therapy practitioners must strive for the inclusion of occupation-based intervention for all clients in order to maximize the client's ability to perform his or her meaningful daily occupations.

Check Your Thinking 3-13

A Adjunctive	E Enabling	P Purposeful	O Occupation-Based
Interventions that prepare for performance and participation	*Interventions that focus on performance skills*	*Interventions that have a pre-determined goal and facilitate practice and problem solving*	*Interventions that are perceived as desirable, match individualized goals, and occur in appropriate context*

Categorize the following list of interventions according to the intervention continuum. The answers can be found in Appendix B.

A = Adjunctive intervention
E = Enabling intervention
P = Purposeful intervention
O = Occupation-based intervention

_____ lifting and carrying a grocery bag filled with occupational therapy clinic food items

_____ fluidotherapy

_____ making chocolate chip cookies in occupational therapy clinic to share with staff and other clients

_____ placing clothespins on a rod

_____ pinch exercises with putty

_____ copying a recipe for a friend

_____ telephoning a grandchild

_____ cutting out coupons collected by the occupational therapy staff

_____ bowling in the clinic

_____ completing self-care tasks in the morning with own adaptive equipment

_____ watering plants in the occupational therapy clinic

_____ making a macramé plant hanger

_____ finishing own latch-hook project brought to the clinic by a family member

_____ transferring from wheelchair to the mat table

_____ purchasing a card for a friend at the gift shop

_____ brushing teeth in the occupational therapy clinic

_____ upper extremity skateboard

_____ reading a self-chosen magazine article when standing at table edge

_____ role-playing a scenario dealing with anger and management techniques

_____ completing a sample check-writing task

A	E	P	O
Adjunctive	**Enabling**	**Purposeful**	**Occupation-Based**
Interventions that prepare for performance and participation	*Interventions that focus on performance skills*	*Interventions that have a predetermined goal and facilitate practice and problem solving*	*Interventions that are perceived as desirable, match individualized goals, and occur in appropriate context*

_____ following a functional ambulation clinic obstacle course with walker

_____ hanging cards received from friends and family in the hospital room with a reacher

_____ verbal education on how to use a reacher

_____ repeated retrieval of objects from the floor using a reacher

_____ wearing a resting hand splint during sleeping hours

_____ use of adaptive equipment when eating breakfast

References

American Occupational Therapy Association. (1979). The philosophical base of Occupational therapy. *American Journal of Occupational Therapy, 33,* 785.

American Occupational Therapy Association. (1993). Position paper: Purposeful activity. *American Journal of Occupational Therapy, 47,* 1081–1082.

American Occupational Therapy Association. (1997). Physical agent modalities: A position paper. *American Journal of Occupational Therapy, 51,* 870–871.

Ayres, A. J. (1958). Basic concepts of clinical practice in physical disabilities. *American Journal of Occupational Therapy, 12,* 300–311.

Bajuk, S., Jelnikar, T., & Ortar, M. (1996). Rehabilitation of patient with brachial plexus lesion and break in axillary artery. *Journal of Hand Therapy, 9,* 399–403.

Chisholm, D., Dolhi, C., & Schreiber, J. (2000a, January 3). Creating occupation-based opportunities in a medical model clinical practice setting. *OT Practice, 5*(1), CE1–8.

Chisholm, D., Dolhi, C., & Schreiber, J. (2000b, June). *Putting occupation where it belongs—In therapy.* Workshop conducted at Kean University, Union, New Jersey.

Clark, F., Azen, S. P., Zemke, R., Jackson, J., Carlson, M., Mandel, D., et al. (1997). Occupational therapy for independent-living older adults: A randomized controlled trial. *Journal of the American Medical Association, 278,* 1321–1326.

Gray, J. M. (1998). Putting occupation into practice: Occupation as ends, occupation as means. *American Journal of Occupational Therapy, 52,* 354–364.

Kleinman, B. L., & Stalcup, A. (1991). The effect of graded craft activities on visuomotor integration in an inpatient child psychiatry population. *American Journal of Occupational Therapy, 50,* 17–23.

Law, M., Baptiste, S., Carswell, A., McColl, M. A., Polatajko, H., & Pollock, N. (1998). *Canadian Occupational Performance Measure* (3rd ed.). Ottowa, Ontario: CAOT Publications ACE.

Maddy, L. S., & Meyerdierks, E. M. (1997). Dynamic extension assist splinting of acute central slip lacerations. *Journal of Hand Therapy, 10,* 206–212.

Pedretti, L. W. (1996a). Occupational performance: A model for practice in physical dysfunction. In L. W. Pedretti (Ed.), *Occupational therapy: Practice skills for physical dysfunction* (4th ed., pp. 3–12). Philadelphia: Mosby.

Pedretti, L. W. (1996b). Use of adjunctive modalities in occupational therapy. In R. P. Fleming-Cottrell (Ed.), *Perspectives on purposeful activity: Foundations and future of occupational therapy* (pp. 451–453). Bethesda, MD: American Occupational Therapy Association.

Pedretti, L. W., & Early, M. B. (2001). Occupational performance and models for practice for physical dysfunction. In L. W. Pedretti & M. B. Early (Eds.), *Occupational therapy: Practice for physical dysfunction* (5th ed., pp. 7–9). St. Louis, MO: Mosby.

Pierce, D. (1998). What is the source of occupation's treatment power? *American Journal of Occupational Therapy, 52,* 490–491.

Suggested Readings

In addition to the references listed in this chapter, the following are useful information sources for interventions.

Fleming, R. P. (Ed.). (1996). *Perspectives on purposeful activity: Foundation and future of occupational therapy.* Bethesda, MD: American Occupational Therapy Association.

Law, M. (2002). Participation in the occupations of everyday life. *American Journal of Occupational Therapy, 56,* 640–649.

Pierce, D. (2001). Occupation by design: Dimensions, therapeutic power, and creative process. *American Journal of Occupational Therapy, 55,* 249–259.

Schell, B. A. B., Crepeau, E. B., & Cohn, E. S. (2003). Overview of intervention. In E. B. Crepeau, E. S. Cohn, & B. A. B. Schell (Eds.), *Willard & Spackman's occupational therapy* (pp. 455–490). Philadelphia: Lippincott Williams & Wilkins.

CHAPTER 4

Practice Analysis

Learning Objectives

After reading this chapter and completing the learning activities, you should be able to do the following:

1. Describe your practice setting and the demographic characteristics of your clients.
2. Identify the areas of occupation, performance skills, performance patterns, and performance contexts you typically address in your clients' occupational therapy intervention plans.
3. Identify examples of the interventions you typically use to address your clients' occupational performance problems in areas of occupation, performance skills, performance patterns, and/or performance contexts.
4. Identify how you use adjunctive, enabling, purposeful, and occupation-based interventions in your clinical practice.
5. Identify circumstances or conditions that facilitate your ability to include occupation-based interventions in your clinical practice.
6. Identify circumstances or conditions that limit your ability to include occupation-based interventions in your clinical practice.

Key Terms and Concepts

practice analysis
areas of occupation
performance skills
performance patterns
performance contexts

INTRODUCTION

The preceding chapters have addressed the use of occupation in occupational therapy practice, a client-centered approach strategy, and the intervention continuum. At this point, we want to focus on *your* clinical practice.

PRACTICE ANALYSIS

Prior to undertaking any change process, it is important to identify and analyze the current situation. Similar to evaluating a client prior to planning and implementing intervention, an analysis assists us in identifying the strengths and problem areas and provides a foundation for decision making. The **practice analysis** is designed to provide you with an opportunity to critically evaluate your current practice. This will assist you in identifying areas where you can increase your use of occupation-based interventions. Each section of the practice analysis is presented separately in order to enhance your understanding of its intent and the relationship between your practice and occupation-based practice. A complete practice analysis is provided in Appendix C for future use.

Practice Analysis—Step 1

Step 1 is designed to help you identify the demographic characteristics of your practice setting and your client population. If you work in a number of different practice settings, it will be useful for you to complete a different practice analysis for each setting. For this step, consider your primary practice setting when responding to the following questions.

What is your occupational therapy practice setting (i.e., acute care, rehabilitation, school system, long-term care, home health, outpatient, etc.)?

What are the typical diagnoses or conditions of your clients?

What is the gender distribution of your clients?

_____ % female

_____ % male

What is the age distribution of your clients?

_____ % birth–3 years

_____ % 4–9 years

_____ % 10–15 years

_____ % 16–21 years

_____ % 22–40 years

_____ % 41–65 years

_____ % 66–80 years

_____ % 80+ years

What are the typical occupational roles of your clients?

What is the average frequency that your clients receive occupational therapy services?

_____ daily

_____ twice daily

_____ # of sessions

_____ other—describe:

What is the average duration that your clients receive occupational therapy services?

_____ 1 week or less

_____ 2–3 weeks

_____ 4–6 weeks

_____ > 6 weeks

_____ other—describe:

What is the typical discharge destination of your clients?

What are the common reimbursement sources for your occupational therapy services?

Practice Analysis—Step 2

In this step you will identify the **areas of occupation**, **performance skills**, **performance patterns**, and/or **performance contexts** that are common problem areas for your clients. Consider your practice setting and the clients you described in Step 1. As you review the occupations, skills, patterns, and contexts in Table 4-1, put a check to the left of the items that are typical problem areas for your clients.

Table 4-1 Areas of Occupation, Performance Skills, Performance Patterns, and Performance Contexts.

✔	AREAS OF OCCUPATION	INTERVENTION	A	E	P	O
	Activities of Daily Living					
	Bathing, showering					
	Bowel and bladder management					
	Dressing					
	Eating					
	Feeding					
	Functional mobility					
	Personal care device					
	Personal hygiene and grooming					
	Sexual activity					
	Sleep/rest					
	Toilet hygiene					
	Instrumental Activities of Daily Living					
	Care of others					
	Care of pets					
	Communication device use					
	Community mobility					
	Financial management					
	Health management and maintenance					

(continues)

| Table 4-1 | Areas of Occupation, Performance Skills, Performance Patterns, and Performance Contexts. *(continued)* | | | | |

✔	AREAS OF OCCUPATION	INTERVENTION	A	E	P	O
	Home establishment and management					
	Meal preparation and clean-up					
	Safety procedures and emergency responses					
	Shopping					
	Education					
	Exploration of informal personal educational needs or interests					
	Formal educational participation					
	Informal personal education participation					
	Work					
	Employment interests and pursuits					
	Employment seeking and acquisition					
	Job performance					
	Retirement preparation and adjustment					
	Volunteer exploration					
	Volunteer participation					
	Play					
	Play exploration					
	Play participation					
	Leisure					
	Leisure exploration					
	Leisure participation					
	Social participation					
	Community					
	Family					

Table 4-1	Areas of Occupation, Performance Skills, Performance Patterns, and Performance Contexts. *(continued)*					

✔	AREAS OF OCCUPATION	INTERVENTION	A	E	P	O
	Peer, friend					
✔	**PERFORMANCE SKILLS**	**INTERVENTION**	A	E	P	O
	Sensorimotor					
	Sensory awareness					
	Sensory processing					
	Tactile					
	Proprioceptive					
	Vestibular					
	Visual					
	Auditory					
	Gustatory					
	Olfactory					
	Perceptual processing					
	Stereognosis					
	Kinesthesia					
	Pain response					
	Body scheme					
	Right/left discrimination					
	Form constancy					
	Position in space					
	Visual-closure					
	Figure ground					
	Depth perception					
	Spatial relations					
	Topographical orientation					
	Neuromusculoskeletal					
	Reflexes					
	Range of motion					
	Muscle tone					

(continues)

Table 4-1	Areas of Occupation, Performance Skills, Performance Patterns, and Performance Contexts. *(continued)*				
✔ **PERFORMANCE SKILLS**	**INTERVENTION**	A	E	P	O
Strength					
Endurance					
Postural control					
Postural alignment					
Soft tissue integrity					
Motor skills					
Gross coordination					
Crossing the midline					
Laterality					
Bilateral integration					
Motor control					
Praxis					
Fine coordination					
Visual-motor integration					
Oral-motor control					
Cognition					
Level of arousal					
Orientation					
Recognition					
Attention span					
Initiation of activity					
Termination of activity					
Memory					
Sequencing					
Categorization					
Concept formation					
Spatial operations					
Problem solving					
Learning					
Generalization					

Table 4-1	Areas of Occupation, Performance Skills, Performance Patterns, and Performance Contexts. *(continued)*				
✔	**PERFORMANCE SKILLS**	**INTERVENTION**	A	E	P	O
	Psychosocial/Psychological					
	Psychological					
	Values					
	Interests					
	Self-concept					
	Social					
	Role performance					
	Social conduct					
	Interpersonal skills					
	Self-expression					
	Self-management					
	Coping skills					
	Time management					
	Self-control					
✔	**PERFORMANCE PATTERNS**	**INTERVENTION**	A	E	P	O
	Habits					
	Routines					
	Roles					
✔	**PERFORMANCE CONTEXTS**	**INTERVENTION**	A	E	P	O
	Cultural					
	Physical					
	Social					
	Personal					
	Spiritual					
	Temporal					
	Virtual					

Note: The areas of occupation, performance patterns, and performance contexts sections are from "Occupational therapy practice framework: Domain and process" by the American Occupational Therapy Association, 2002, *American Journal of Occupational Therapy, 56,* 620–623. Copyright 2002 by the American Occupational Therapy Association, Inc. Adapted with permission. The performance skills section is from the rescinded "Uniform terminology for occupational therapy—third edition" by the American Occupational Therapy Association, 1994, *American Journal of Occupational Therapy, 48,* 1047–1054. Copyright 1994 by the American Occupational Therapy Association, Inc. Adapted with permission.

Practice Analysis—Step 3

Consider the practice setting and clients you described in Step 1. Return to Table 4-1 and identify an example(s) of an intervention that you typically use to address the problem occupations, skills, patterns, or contexts you checked. Write your example(s) in the column titled "Intervention." You are encouraged to write more than one example if you typically use more than one type of intervention to address the problem.

Practice Analysis—Step 4

Having completed the first three steps of the practice analysis, you now have a global picture of your practice setting, your clients, their problem occupations, skills, patterns, and contexts, and the interventions you typically use to address their problems.

The next step in analyzing your practice is to categorize the interventions you include in your clients' occupational therapy intervention plans. For Step 4, return to the interventions you wrote in Table 4-1. As you review each intervention try to recall a "real life" clinical situation when you used the intervention with one of your clients. How would you categorize the intervention, from your "real life" clinical situation, in the intervention continuum presented in Chapter 3? Is it an adjunctive intervention? Is it an enabling intervention? Is it a purposeful intervention? Or is it an occupation-based intervention? Place a check mark in the box to the right of your intervention that you feel best represents the category of the intervention—A = adjunctive intervention; E = enabling intervention; P = purposeful intervention; and O = occupation-based intervention. The definitions and examples provided in Chapter 3 can help you identify the appropriate intervention category. Remember that many interventions reflect more than one category, so choose the category that best defines how you use that intervention in your clinical practice.

After completing Step 4, examine the distribution of your interventions within the categories of the continuum. Consider the following questions:

1. Are the interventions that you listed evenly distributed across the categories of the continuum?

2. Do you use more (or less) adjunctive interventions than other types of interventions?

3. Do you use more (or less) enabling interventions than other types of interventions?

4. Do you use more (or less) purposeful interventions than other types of interventions?

5. Do you use more (or less) occupation-based interventions than other types of interventions?

6. Which type of intervention do you use the most?

7. Which type of intervention do you use the least?

Practice Analysis—Step 5

It is not uncommon for practitioners to use more than one intervention to address a specific occupation, performance skill, pattern, or context. As previously stated, many interventions can reflect more than one category of the intervention continuum and some interventions can cross categories depending on how and why they are implemented. The selection of an intervention depends on a variety of client, practitioner, and setting factors. For example, Barb, a mother of three children, with fibromyalgia may need, want, and be expected to perform home management tasks. You choose work simplification strategies as an intervention to improve her ability to perform home management tasks. However, Barb's current level of activity performance prevents her from getting out of bed, so you provide her with written information on work simplification techniques that she can review on her own. Providing Barb with written materials is an adjunctive intervention. As Barb's activity performance status improves, you may have her use the work simplification techniques while preparing chocolate chip cookies in the occupational therapy clinic to give to her children when they visit. This situation moves the intervention to the occupation-based category of the continuum. In this example, the acuity of Barb's condition impacted the choice of intervention.

Duration of services and practice setting may also influence the interventions you use with a client. Consider Martin, a retired steelworker, who had a total knee replacement and is being discharged to his home from the acute care hospital two days post-surgery. While intervention protocols related to Martin's condition frequently focus on enhancing independence and safety in self-care and mobility activities, the amount of time available to instruct Martin in the use of adaptive equipment to perform self-care activities is limited. This situation could be further complicated if Martin's wife is unable to be involved in his therapy program, or if Martin does not have his own clothes and supplies at the hospital, or your schedule restricts you to seeing Martin in the occupational therapy clinic. In these situations, it may be necessary for you to use more enabling and/or purposeful interventions in Martin's therapy program such as demonstrating the use of equipment, discussing options for obtaining the equipment, using the equipment in simulated situations, and /or identifying and problem solving potential safety hazards that Martin may encounter at home.

In these two examples, the degree of acuity, length of stay, and practice setting context impacted the practitioner's choice of interventions. Additionally, other factors such as client preference, availability of supplies, space, and/or scheduling demands can affect your choice of an intervention.

Step 5 will help you examine the range of interventions you routinely use or could use in your clinical practice. For example, Box 4-1 illustrates that interventions addressing an area of occupation can span the categories of the continuum. Each description represents a potentially appropriate occupational therapy intervention for reducing a client's area of occupation deficit (dressing) depending on the specifics of the client and practice setting. The intervention examples are not meant to reflect best practice, but are designed to provide guidance for the development of interventions for this area of occupation. The occupational therapy practitioner is responsible for using clinical judgment regarding the appropriateness of any given intervention as determined by a specific client's circumstances.

BOX 4-1   **Intervention Examples for an Area of Occupation**

Areas of Occupation	EXAMPLES			
	Adjunctive	**Enabling**	**Purposeful**	**Occupation-Based**
Dressing	Written material on one-handed dressing techniques	Practicing buttoning using a button aid and a dressing board	Donning and doffing a button-down shirt that belongs to the occupational therapy department over client's clothing during an afternoon therapy session	Donning a button-down shirt and using a button aid to fasten the buttons—all as part of the client's morning self-care in his or her hospital room

Referring back to Step 2, identify a common area of occupation, performance skill, performance pattern, or performance context that you typically address in your clients' therapy programs. Consider the interventions that you use or could use to address the occupation, skill, pattern, and/or context problem across the continuum categories. Boxes 4-2 through 4-5 provide you with the opportunity to complete this exercise for a range of occupations, performance skills, performance patterns, and performance contexts. Identifying a range of interventions can help you to develop interventions that span the continuum categories. It can also facilitate your growth as an occupation-based practitioner.

BOX 4-2   Intervention Exercise: Areas of Occupation

Areas of Occupation	EXAMPLES			
	A Adjunctive	**E** Enabling	**P** Purposeful	**O** Occupation-Based

BOX 4-3   Intervention Exercise: Performance Skills

Performance Skills	EXAMPLES			
	A Adjunctive	**E** Enabling	**P** Purposeful	**O** Occupation-Based

BOX 4-4 Intervention Exercise: Performance Patterns

Performance Patterns	EXAMPLES			
	Adjunctive	Enabling	Purposeful	Occupation-Based

BOX 4-5 Intervention Exercise: Performance Contexts

Performance Contexts	EXAMPLES			
	Adjunctive	Enabling	Purposeful	Occupation-Based

Practice Analysis—Step 6

Step 6, the final step in the practice analysis, requires that you look beyond the direct services of your occupational therapy practice. In this step you will identify the issues that impact your ability to use occupation-based interventions in your day-to-day practice. These issues might be related to the environment, equipment and supplies, treatment space, administrative support, caseload demands, and/or documentation requirements, to name a few. You will be generating two lists of issues. One list will include those issues that positively influence or facilitate your ability to include occupation-based interventions in your clients' therapy programs. The other list will include those issues that negatively impact or restrict your use of occupation-based interventions. Consider adding to these lists as you identify additional issues or as new issues arise. In addition, we encourage you to start a "wish list" that includes those "wishes" that, if you had them, would help you to provide occupation-based interventions more consistently.

➤ What circumstances or issues facilitate your ability to include occupation-based interventions in your clients' therapy programs?

[blank response box]

➤ What circumstances or issues limit your ability to use occupation-based interventions in your clinical practice?

[blank response box]

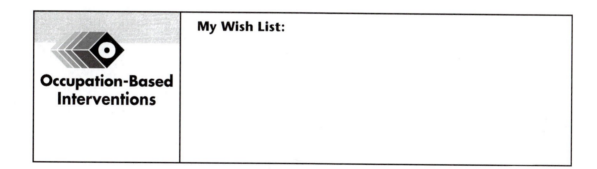

Occupation-Based Interventions | **My Wish List:**

Summary

Analyzing your current practice is an essential preliminary step to facilitate your professional competence in maximizing the use of occupation in your clients' intervention plans. Upon completing the practice analysis for your practice setting, you should have a clear understanding of your clients' demographic profiles and their occupational performance deficits. In addition, you should have an increased awareness of the interventions that you commonly use and how they relate to the intervention continuum. This insight about your current practice, combined with your knowledge of the intervention continuum, will facilitate your development as an occupation-based practitioner.

References

American Occupational Therapy Association. (1994). Uniform terminology for occupational therapy—third edition. *American Journal of Occupational Therapy, 48,* 1047–1054.

American Occupational Therapy Association. (2002). Occupational therapy practice framework: Domain and process. *American Journal of Occupational Therapy, 56,* 609–639.

Suggested Readings

In addition to the references listed in this chapter, the following are useful information sources for analyzing your practice.

Lewin, J. E., & Reed, C. A. (1998). *Creative problem solving in occupational therapy.* Philadelphia: Lippincott-Raven Publishers.

Mandel, D. R., Jackson, J. M, Zemke, R., Nelson, L., & Clark, F. A. (1999). Needs evaluation. *Lifestyle redesign: Implementing the well elderly program.* Bethesda, MD: American Occupational Therapy Association.

Schell, B. A. B. (2003). Clinical reasoning: The basis of practice. In E. B. Crepeau, E. S. Cohn, & B. A. B. Schell (Eds.), *Willard & Spackman's occupational therapy* (pp. 131–139). Philadelphia: Lippincott Williams & Wilkins.

CHAPTER 5

Obstacles and Opportunities

Learning Objectives

After reading this chapter and completing the learning activities, you should be able to do the following:

1. Identify assets or opportunities that can facilitate the use of occupation-based interventions in your clinical practice.
2. Identify obstacles that restrict the use of occupation-based interventions in your clinical practice.
3. Develop a plan of action for transitioning obstacles into occupation-based practice opportunities.

Key Terms and Concepts

obstacles
opportunities
assets
space
caseload
supplies and equipment
administration
clients
interdisciplinary team
documentation
reimbursement
time
budget
occupational therapy practitioners

INTRODUCTION

As part of the practice analysis in Chapter 4, you identified circumstances or conditions that you feel affect your ability to provide occupation-based practice. Take a moment and return to Step 6 of *your* practice analysis and review the issues that you identified as limiting your ability to include occupation-based interventions in your clinical practice. Since most practitioners are not in a position to simply remove their practice **obstacles**, it is necessary to transition the obstacles into **opportunities**.

In this chapter, we provide you with ideas for transforming the obstacles that are hindering your use of occupation-based practice into opportunities. Practitioners have informed us that many of these ideas were helpful to them when they were faced with similar obstacles as they struggled and worked toward enhancing their occupation-based practice. Every idea will not work for every practitioner or in every clinical setting, and some of the ideas may be effective for managing more than one obstacle. The ideas are not intended to be prescriptive, restrictive, or all inclusive. Clearly, some of the ideas will be easier to implement than others, as some obstacles are more amenable to change. Our list of ideas is intended to provide you with a starting point from which you can generate your own ideas for transforming your practice obstacles into opportunities.

To help you do so, it will be important to develop a plan of action. First, you will need to identify your current **assets** or opportunities—the things that do or can assist you in being an occupation-based practitioner. Next you will need to identify the obstacles in your clinical practice. And finally, you will need to identify ideas for transitioning each obstacle into an occupation-based practice opportunity. Your list of assets, in conjunction with the ideas we have provided, can be helpful in developing your plan of action. In this chapter you will develop a plan of action for each clinical practice issue. Recognizing the obstacle is the first step in identifying possible solutions. After you have developed your plan of action for each issue, prioritize the obstacles and implement your action plans starting with the most pressing obstacles, or those easiest to transition into an opportunity, or those that have guaranteed success. Remember, it will take time to transition your obstacles into opportunities. And as part of the process you may have to trial and modify solutions in order to find the one that works for your situation. Good luck—we know you can do it.

SPACE

Many occupational therapy practitioners have told us that physical **space** limits their ability to engage their clients in occupation-based interventions. If this sounds familiar to you, ask yourself what it is about your clinical space that is problematic. Take a critical look at your clinical space and consider the following questions:

➤ Do you have a space dedicated for occupational therapy services?

➤ Is your clinic space the right size?

➤ Do you have the right kind of furniture?

➤ Are you and your clients able to use the space effectively?

Make a list of the assets related to your space.

Make a list of the obstacles related to your space.

Now consider the following space ideas:

➤ Look around your facility and determine if there are "spaces" better suited to your clients' needs. One of the most obvious options in an inpatient setting is the client's room in the facility. Other commonly identified alternatives that support occupation-based practice include public lounges, vending machine areas, gift shops, visitor restrooms, pay phones, cafeterias, chapels, and pantries or kitchens typically used by staff or family members.

➤ Carefully consider the occupations and performance skills, patterns, and contexts being addressed in a client's intervention plan. Can these areas be addressed as part of transporting the client to the occupational therapy area? If so, begin the intervention session at the client's room, a building entrance, or at the location of the client's prior appointment so that the transport time becomes part of the intervention session, thereby maximizing your time and space.

➤ While it is often helpful to see clients who have similar occupational performance needs at the same time, it may not be feasible if they all need to use the same equipment/furniture/space. Consider rearranging the clients' therapy schedules so that your space is used optimally.

➤ Consider the feasibility of exchanging space with another discipline/department. You may find that another discipline/department is experiencing similar challenges with their space and that the exchange would meet both of your needs.

➤ Determine your space needs for implementing occupation-based interventions. Be realistic. Justify and document them. Then, determine if and when capital renovations are being planned and make your needs known.

Now develop your space plan of action.

SPACE OBSTACLE

_____
_____
_____
_____

SPACE OPPORTUNITY

_____
_____
_____
_____

CASELOAD

Have you ever thought to yourself "so many patients, so little time"? If so, your thinking is the same as many of your colleagues. Practitioners frequently identify high **caseload** volumes, high acuity levels, and multiple demands on their time as obstacles to implementing occupation-based interventions. Critically think about your caseload and consider the following questions:

➤ What is the typical number of clients on your caseload?
➤ Does your caseload represent a wide or narrow range of diagnoses/conditions?
➤ What is the acuity level of your clients?
➤ What are the demands associated with your caseload?

Make a list of the assets related to your caseload.

Make a list of the obstacles related to your caseload.

```



```

Now consider the following caseload ideas:

➤ Think about the occupational performance needs of your clients and the impairments that contribute to their occupational performance deficits. Scheduling clients who have similar needs during the same session can be an effective strategy for treating more than one client at a time. The key for making this approach successful is to ensure that clients who are grouped together have comparable skill levels and complementary occupational needs. An additional advantage to this approach is that clients are afforded the opportunity to interact with others who are experiencing similar occupational performance challenges. Remember to check your reimbursement regulations.

➤ Consider the use of group treatment. Careful planning can facilitate successful, meaningful group interventions. Plan ahead for occupation-based intervention groups by identifying the goals to be accomplished by the group, criteria for participation including skills needed by group members to engage in the intervention, and the required supplies and equipment. Planning will help you avoid rushing at the last minute and will enable you to focus on the intervention and the clients' responses to it. Group development is an excellent student project since it requires the coordination and implementation of a number of skills that students need to develop. Using a template (see Appendix D) for group development and storing the associated supplies and equipment in a labeled storage container will make it easier to implement the group intervention and will save you time. Remember to check your reimbursement regulations.

➤ Critically analyze the frequency and duration patterns of your caseload. Provide each client with what he or she needs and will benefit from—no more and no less.

➤ Develop and maintain strong working relationships with all of the members of your occupational therapy team, including therapists, assistants, and aides. Determine how each team member can contribute most effectively to enhancing your team's use of occupation-based practice.

➤ Adjunctive and enabling interventions can be appropriately used to help you manage multiple clients within the same intervention session. Remember that these interventions should be linked with the client's priority occupations.

Now develop your caseload plan of action.

CASELOAD OBSTACLE   **CASELOAD OPPORTUNITY**

_____   _____

_____   _____

_____   _____

_____   _____

SUPPLIES AND EQUIPMENT

One of the most frustrating situations that occupational therapy practitioners face occurs when they have a great idea for a treatment intervention that will ideally meet a client's occupational performance needs, only to find that the required **supplies and equipment** are not available. This seemingly small frustration may be perceived as an insurmountable obstacle if it happens repeatedly. Critically think about your clinical supplies and equipment and consider the following questions:

➤ What clinical supplies and equipment do you have readily available?

➤ Do your supplies and equipment meet the occupational performance needs of your clients?

➤ Are there supplies and equipment in your clinic that you don't use? If so, why?

➤ What supplies and equipment do you wish were available?

Make a list of the assets related to your supplies and equipment.

Make a list of the obstacles related to your supplies and equipment.

Now consider the following supplies and equipment ideas:

➤ Once again, planning is essential. In order to be prepared, identify the supplies and equipment you commonly use in practice. One way to do this is to refer back to your practice analysis and reflect on the demographic information that you reported. Consider your clients' occupational profiles. This step will help you to brainstorm possible interventions that will complement your clients' needs in order to determine the required supplies and equipment.

➤ After you have identified supplies and equipment that you use and need, take an inventory of what is currently available in your clinic (don't forget to look in drawers and in the back of the closets). If your supply and equipment budget is adequate, purchase the supplies and equipment that you need. Since many of the supplies and equipment needed for implementing occupation-based interventions are those that people routinely use in their daily lives, there are other options for obtaining supplies and equipment. With your clients in mind, think about the following approaches for obtaining what you need:

- Clean your (or your neighbor's) closets, cupboards, and drawers. Items that may no longer be of use to you or others in your home may be the supplies or equipment required for occupation-based interventions.

- Go to flea markets, garage sales, discount stores, or local shops that sell used clothing and household goods to purchase items that can supplement your supply and equipment inventory.

- Look for free samples of products—your clients can use the samples (e.g., cosmetics, cologne, or products from conference exhibit halls) as part of their intervention program.

- Maintain a collection of the following:
  - coupons, catalogs, and junk mail;
  - coins and coin wrappers;
  - gift boxes and wrapping paper;
  - grocery bags; and
  - an assortment of canned and boxed goods

- Organize a "drive" in your facility during Occupational Therapy Month to collect items that you need. Use this event as an opportunity to explain occupational therapy and occupation-based interventions.

- Have the students assigned to your facility develop intervention kits (i.e., a kit might include supplies and equipment needed for manicuring, sewing, carpentry, crossword or word search puzzles, etc.).

- Speak with the volunteer department in your facility, church groups, and/or community service organizations and ask them to assist you in collecting the supplies and equipment that you need.

- Ask your client's family or caregivers to bring supplies and equipment that the client uses from his or her home. Using the client's own clothing and objects maximizes the occupation-based nature of intervention.

Now develop your supplies and equipment plan of action.

SUPPLIES AND EQUIPMENT OBSTACLE   SUPPLIES AND EQUIPMENT OPPORTUNITY

_____   _____

_____   _____

_____   _____

_____   _____

ADMINISTRATION

Some practitioners have told us that a lack of support from their **administration** restricts their ability to provide occupation-based interventions. This lack of support may be caused by a lack of understanding about the domain and process of occupational therapy practice. Presuming that to be the case, it is our responsibility as occupational therapy practitioners to educate the administrators in our facility. We need to educate them about the domain of our profession so that they understand our unique focus on occupation, what occupation is, and how occupation-based interventions facilitate our clients' participation in their life situations. Critically think about your administration and consider the following questions:

➤ Does my administration understand the unique focus of occupational therapy?

➤ Have I educated my administration about the domain and process of occupational therapy?

➤ Is my administration aware of the supplies and equipment needed to provide occupation-based practice?

➤ Do I have access to and utilize evidence (research) that supports the efficacy of occupational therapy services?

Make a list of the assets related to your administration.

Make a list of the obstacles related to your administration.

```
```

Now consider the following administration ideas:

➤ Seek administrative support inside and outside of your occupational therapy department.

➤ Read and circulate literature that supports occupation-based practice to the administration.

➤ Offer to serve on facility and community committees and task forces where your unique training will be demonstrated and utilized (e.g., safety committee, community rebuilding projects) and where occupation is relevant and meaningful (e.g., special events committee).

➤ Measure and examine your clients' outcomes (e.g., occupational performance, client satisfaction, role competence, adaptation, health and wellness, prevention, quality of life) and share the results with your colleagues and administrators. This is a great student project.

➤ In addition to sharing your findings with your colleagues and administrators in your facility, look for opportunities to publish your results so that other occupational therapy practitioners can benefit from your findings.

Now develop your administration plan of action.

ADMINISTRATION OBSTACLE	ADMINISTRATION OPPORTUNITY

CLIENTS

A satisfied client goes a long way. This is especially true if your satisfied **clients** understand how occupational therapy services can facilitate their ability to engage in meaningful occupations that, in turn, support participation in their lives. If your clients do not understand the unique role of occupational therapy, even the positive effects of occupation-based interventions can be negated. Critically think about your clients and consider the following questions:

➤ Have I educated my clients about the unique focus, domain, and process of occupational therapy?

➤ Are my clients aware of how occupational therapy interventions facilitate engagement in their occupations to support participation in their lives?

➤ Have I shared the evidence (research) that supports occupational therapy intervention with my clients?

➤ Have I adequately explained to the client, from an occupation-based perspective, the rationale and purpose of each intervention?

Make a list of the assets related to your clients.

```
┌─────────────────────────────────────────────────────┐
│                                                       │
│                                                       │
│                                                       │
│                                                       │
│                                                       │
│                                                       │
└─────────────────────────────────────────────────────┘
```

Make a list of the obstacles related to your clients.

```
┌─────────────────────────────────────────────────────┐
│                                                       │
│                                                       │
│                                                       │
│                                                       │
└─────────────────────────────────────────────────────┘
```

Now consider the following client ideas:

➤ Think about how you define occupational therapy to your clients. Practice describing occupational therapy to people unfamiliar with the profession. Use terminology and examples they can relate to and understand. Use the word "occupation"—and use it frequently. Include examples of your client's occupations in your description.

➤ Avoid introducing yourself to your clients as "Joe (or Jane) from OT." Introduce yourself as an "occupational therapist," "occupational therapy assistant," or "occupational therapy student" and then describe how your skilled services (i.e., occupational therapy) may benefit him or her.

➤ Talk about "occupation" with clients and their significant others. Use each contact as an opportunity to describe and reinforce the power and value of occupation.

➤ Maximize the client-centered approach. Solicit your clients' input about their goals and interventions and incorporate their input in their therapy program. If you are unable to address a goal or include a certain intervention, explain the reason to the client.

➤ Give your clients as many intervention choices as possible to facilitate their input and commitment to their therapy program.

➤ Encourage satisfied clients and/or their families to share their occupational therapy experience with your administration in the form of a letter or a face-to-face meeting.

Now develop your client plan of action.

CLIENT OBSTACLE

_____

_____

_____

_____

CLIENT OPPORTUNITY

_____

_____

_____

_____

INTERDISCIPLINARY TEAM

Have you ever had a member of your **interdisciplinary team** say, "his arms work, he doesn't really need occupational therapy" or "she has too much free time in her schedule—send her to occupational therapy for something to do"? These and similar statements are clear evidence that the speaker does not fully understand the role of occupational therapy. In order for other health care professionals to appropriately refer clients for occupational therapy services and seek out our expertise, it is essential that these professionals understand and value occupation and its application in the intervention process. Critically think about the members of your interdisciplinary team and support staff, and consider the following questions:

➤ Have I educated my interdisciplinary team about the domain and process of occupational therapy?

➤ Do my interdisciplinary team members understand how engagement in occupation supports our clients' participation in their life situations?

➤ Is my interdisciplinary team aware of how occupational therapy interventions can facilitate engagement in occupation to support our clients' participation in their lives?

➤ Have I shared the evidence (research) that supports occupational therapy services with my interdisciplinary team?

Make a list of the assets related to your interdisciplinary team.

Make a list of the obstacles related to your interdisciplinary team.

Now consider the following interdisciplinary team ideas:

➤ Develop a clear and concise professional description of occupational therapy that focuses on occupation and is appropriate for the context of the services provided by your interdisciplinary team.

➤ Conduct innovative celebrations for Occupational Therapy Month. One practitioner provided her colleagues with the opportunity to complete their own client-centered interview and apply their results by completing a "Pie of Life" chart (N. Speakman, personal communication, July 11, 2002). The chart helped illustrate how they were using their time. At the end of the activity, participants were given a piece of "pie" and a handout describing the role of occupational therapy in that practice setting.

➤ Co-treat with other disciplines and demonstrate how the use of occupation-based interventions can positively influence a client's performance.

➤ Obtain and share literature including the results of evidence-based (research) studies that support the use of occupation-based interventions in practice settings similar to yours. (Evidence will be discussed in Chapter 6.)

➤ Provide an in-service to your interdisciplinary team that identifies the power and importance of occupation in their lives and the lives of their clients. Follow it up with a real-life case study from your caseload that illustrates the application of occupation-based intervention to enhance the client's participation in life.

Now develop your interdisciplinary team plan of action.

INTERDISCIPLINARY TEAM OBSTACLE	INTERDISCIPLINARY TEAM OPPORTUNITY
_____	_____
_____	_____
_____	_____
_____	_____

DOCUMENTATION

Documentation is often considered a necessary evil. Documentation serves many purposes including those related to program evaluation, clinical outcomes, reimbursement, requirements of regulatory agencies, and legal considerations. Critically look at and think about your documentation and consider the following questions:

➤ What is my documentation process—how, when, what, and where do I document?

➤ Does my documentation focus on the client's performance of occupations, or does it only address skill performance impairments?

➤ Does my documentation include occupational performance outcomes?

➤ Does my documentation reflect the occupation-based interventions used with the client?

Make a list of the assets related to your documentation.

Make a list of the obstacles related to your documentation.

Now consider the following documentation ideas:

➤ Carefully review and analyze your documentation forms. Determine if they appropriately reflect occupational therapy's unique focus on occupation.

➤ Don't duplicate the documentation of other disciplines. Use your documentation to focus on the client's progress toward engagement in occupation.

➤ Be sure that you have accurate information about documentation requirements. Find out what is required and by whom. It is not uncommon for practitioners to fall prey to "we've always done it that way" without identifying the reason it is done that way or determining its appropriateness in the ever-changing world of health care. Third-party payers typically want information indicating what a client can do and whether the client is safe doing it—both of which focus on engagement in occupation.

➤ If necessary, revise your documentation forms.
  • Use checklists whenever possible to decrease the amount of time spent writing, as long as using the checklist does not minimize the use of occupation-based interventions.
  • Use the "Occupational Therapy Practice Framework: Domain and Process" (American Occupational Therapy Association, 2002) and relevant occupational therapy models of practice to guide your documentation.
  • Make every form and word count—focus on quality versus quantity. Make recommendations to your supervisor for streamlining your documentation process.

➤ Use the word "occupation" in your documentation (and discussions) instead of "activity" or "task," and provide examples of your client's occupations.

➤ Be sure that your goals reflect the client's engagement in occupation. Highlight the occupational performance or occupation outcome.

Now develop your documentation plan of action.

DOCUMENTATION OBSTACLE   **DOCUMENTATION OPPORTUNITY**

_____   _____

_____   _____

_____   _____

_____   _____

REIMBURSEMENT

Many practitioners refrain from using occupation-based interventions based on misperceptions that occupation-based services will not be reimbursed. It is critical for occupational therapy practitioners to be knowledgeable of applicable

reimbursement structures. Critically think about your reimbursement sources and consider the following questions:

➤ Who pays for the occupational therapy services I provide?

➤ Do I understand the reimbursement guidelines in my facility?

➤ Who can assist me in becoming more knowledgeable about my reimbursement structure and its guidelines?

➤ Do I have or can I access the evidence (research) that supports the reimbursement of occupational therapy services?

Make a list of the assets related to your reimbursement.

Make a list of the obstacles related to your reimbursement.

Now consider the following reimbursement ideas:

➤ Become familiar with the billing codes used by payers in your practice setting.

➤ Take the initiative to determine the payers' reimbursement requirements and guidelines.

➤ Become familiar with the Current Procedural Terminology (CPT) codes relevant to occupational therapy services (American Medical Association, 2002).

➤ Use the practice guidelines published by the American Occupational Therapy Association to gain a greater understanding of the CPT codes as they relate to specific diagnostic groups.

➤ Use the American Occupational Therapy Association Guide to Occupational Therapy Practice (Moyers, 1999) as a reference for linking occupational therapy evaluation and intervention with billing codes.

➤ Avoid getting caught in the "they won't pay for it, so I can't do it" trap. It is the professional responsibility of occupational therapy practitioners to advocate for the needs of their clients and for the contributions of occupational therapy.

➤ Be an active member in state and national associations—use state and national association resources to obtain reimbursement information and identify ways that you can affect positive change to facilitate reimbursement of occupational therapy services.

➤ Be knowledgeable of legislation that affects occupational therapy services. Read it, understand it, and take action. Your state and national associations are great resources.

Now develop your reimbursement plan of action.

REIMBURSEMENT OBSTACLE

_____

_____

_____

_____

REIMBURSEMENT OPPORTUNITY

_____

_____

_____

_____

TIME

"I don't have enough time." "There isn't enough time." "That takes too much time." Sound familiar? Practitioners often use **time** as a reason for not providing occupation-based practice. Time can be categorized into one (or more) of the following: evaluation time, planning time, and intervention time. The key to having enough time is to maximize the time you do have. Critically think about your time and consider the following questions:

➤ How much time do I spend on tasks related to evaluation? Planning or preparation? Intervention?

➤ Do I maximize the time I spend with clients facilitating their engagement in occupation?

➤ How much time do I spend on nonbillable tasks?

➤ If I had more time in my day, what would I do with it?

Make a list of the assets related to your time.

Make a list of the obstacles related to your time.

Now consider the following time ideas:

➤ Use the occupation-based treatment kits and groups that you had students develop to help you manage more than one client at a time while implementing occupation-based intervention.

➤ Some of the best intervention ideas often come at the most inopportune time—while you are taking a shower or driving home from work. Put a pad and pencil on your nightstand or on the sink in your bathroom; carry a handheld tape recorder and make verbal notes to yourself in the car when stopped at a traffic light; or call and leave a message for yourself on your home or work answering machine.

➤ Use a top-down approach to client evaluation by focusing on areas of occupation and contexts first and then more thoroughly evaluating only the skills and impairments that are restricting the client's occupational performance.

➤ Use a client-centered approach and actively engage the client throughout the occupational therapy process. By doing so, you not only focus on what is important to the client but also use your time more effectively.

➤ Utilize all levels of occupational therapy personnel wisely—from therapists, to therapy assistants, to aides/technicians.

Now develop your time plan of action.

TIME OBSTACLE

TIME OPPORTUNITY

BUDGET

Budget restrictions and the resulting difficulty in obtaining the supplies and equipment needed for occupation-based practice is an obstacle for many occupational therapy practitioners. Since occupation-based practice is focused on the occupations of daily life, the materials needed to perform those occupations are readily available in our day-to-day lives. A well-supplied occupational therapy clinic will reflect the occupational profiles and needs of its clients. This is an opportunity for you to be creative. Critically think about your budget and consider the following questions:

➤ What is my budget and who controls or directs the budget and its development?

➤ Have I identified the supplies and equipment needed to provide occupation-based practice for my client population?

➤ Does the budget allocation reflect the purchase of supplies and equipment needed for occupation-based practice?

➤ What is included in my budget wish list?

Make a list of the assets related to your budget.

Make a list of the obstacles related to your budget.

Now consider the following budget ideas:

➤ Speak with the purchasing agent for your facility to determine which vendors or manufacturers are willing to provide your clinic with trial equipment.

➤ Talk to local vendors about obtaining equipment on a permanent loan basis for use in your clinic.

➤ Arrange for vendors to provide an in-service to your department on new equipment or supplies. Request sample or loaner items, with the understanding that you will use them with your clients and provide the vendor with feedback related to the clients' degree of satisfaction and a summary of the effectiveness of the equipment.

➤ If you are in need of a large piece of equipment, do a financial analysis of the cost benefit that the organization will recoup if the equipment is purchased.

➤ Identify supplies that you could use with your clients that are currently not in use (look in closets and storage areas).

➤ Borrow equipment from other departments (e.g., if a patient needs to practice shoveling or mowing the grass, contact the staff in the physical plant and maintenance department).

➤ Identify potential grant funding sources. This is a great student project, and educational programs are an excellent resource in getting starting.

Now develop your budget plan of action.

BUDGET OBSTACLE

_____

_____

_____

_____

BUDGET OPPORTUNITY

_____

_____

_____

_____

OCCUPATIONAL THERAPY PRACTITIONERS

We've talked about everyone else involved with your practice—the interdisciplinary team, the client, the payers, the administrators—what about you and your colleagues—**occupational therapy practitioners**? Unfortunately, we have found that occupational therapy practitioners often minimize the value and power of occupation. Each and every practitioner is responsible for the advancement of occupational therapy. We must understand, believe in, and communicate our unique focus on occupation. But, we must not be "all talk and no action"—we must use occupation-based interventions in our practice. The old adage "seeing is believing" is true. It is up to occupational therapy practitioners, all of us, to demonstrate how occupation is influential in health and quality of life. Critically think about yourself and other occupational therapy practitioners and consider the following questions:

➤ Do I (they) understand the unique focus of occupational therapy?

➤ Can I (they) articulate the domain and process of occupational therapy in a clear and concise manner?

➤ Do I (they) support occupation-based practice in what I (they) say and do?

➤ Do I (they) have and use evidence (research) on the efficacy of occupational therapy services and/or occupation-based practice?

➤ Am I an effective role model for my profession?

Make a list of the assets related to you and your colleagues.

Make a list of the obstacles related to you and your colleagues.

Now consider the following occupational therapy practitioner ideas:

➤ Read the literature that impacts your practice and your profession.

➤ Schedule a lunchtime or after-work journal club to discuss professional literature with your colleagues.

➤ Invite the faculty from colleges and universities in your area to participate in a journal club or present an evidence-based in-service.

➤ Be knowledgeable of and involved in the efforts of your local, state, and national occupational therapy professional organizations.

➤ Find a mentor (or be one)—having someone that you trust and respect with whom you can discuss current practice issues is invaluable to your professional growth and development.

➤ Join an electronic listserv that addresses your practice issues. Contact your local, state, and/or national occupational therapy associations as resources.

➤ Attend continuing education sessions that address your practice issues or request specific topics to be included at conferences or local state association meetings.

Now develop your occupational therapy practitioner plan of action.

OCCUPATIONAL THERAPY PRACTITIONER OBSTACLE

_____
_____
_____
_____

OCCUPATIONAL THERAPY PRACTITIONER OPPORTUNITY

_____
_____
_____
_____

OTHER ISSUES

Your specific practice setting may have other issues that affect your ability to incorporate occupation-based practice.

Make a list of the assets related to other issues.

```



```

Make a list of the obstacles related to other issues.

```



```

Now develop your other issues plan of action.

OTHER OBSTACLES

_____
_____
_____
_____

OTHER OPPORTUNITIES

_____
_____
_____
_____

Summary

We've covered many issues in this chapter. We hope that the information has sparked excitement and ideas for promoting both occupational therapy and occupation-based practice. It has been our experience that occupational therapy practitioners are individuals who not only enjoy but also take pride in what they do. So, take a few of the suggestions presented in this chapter and put some of your plans into action. Go for it!

References

American Medical Association. (2002). *Current procedural terminology: CPT 2003.* Chicago, IL: Author.

American Occupational Therapy Association. (2002). Occupational therapy practice framework: Domain and process. *American Journal of Occupational Therapy, 56,* 609–639.

Moyers, P. (1999). The guide to occupational therapy practice. *American Journal of Occupational Therapy, 53,* 247–322.

Suggested Readings

In addition to the references listed in this chapter, the following are useful information sources for transitioning obstacles into opportunities for occupation-based practice.

American Occupational Therapy Association. (2002). *Practice guidelines series—complete set.* Bethesda, MD: Author.

Holst, C., & Vogt, D. (1999). *Empowering occupational therapy.* Columbia, MO: TheraPower LLC.

CHAPTER 6

Presenting the Evidence

Learning Objectives

After reading this chapter and completing the learning activities, you should be able to do the following:

1. Understand the need for evidence-based practice in occupational therapy.
2. Identify strategies and keywords for performing literature searches that are relevant to your clinical practice and occupation-based practice.
3. Classify the interventions presented in evidence-based articles as being adjunctive, enabling, purposeful, or occupation-based interventions.

Key Terms and Concepts

occupation-based practice
evidence-based practice

INTRODUCTION

Occupational therapy practitioners' struggle to define and measure occupation has contributed to our restricted progress over the years in generating the evidence that supports and validates our profession. Although public and professional awareness of occupational therapy seems to have increased, the challenge of being considered a profession based on evidence that validates **occupation-based practice** continues. Experts describe **evidence-based practice** as follows:

➤ ". . . care that takes place when decisions that affect the care of patients are taken with due weight accorded to all valid, relevant information" (Hicks as cited in Bury & Mead, 1998, p. 4).

➤ ". . . an approach to decision making in which the clinician uses the best evidence available, in consultation with the patient, to decide upon the option which suits that patient best" (Muir Gray as cited in Law, 2002, p. 9).

➤ ". . . represents the fundamental principle that the provision of quality care will depend on our ability to make choices that have been confirmed by sound scientific data, and that our decisions are based on the best evidence currently available" (Portney & Watkins, 2000, p. 3).

➤ ". . . the integration of best research evidence (clinically relevant research) with clinical expertise and patient values" (Sackett, Straus, Richardson, Rosenberg, & Haynes, 2000, p. 1).

Providing empirical evidence that supports the effectiveness of services is a challenge that all practitioners must accept. The public and the health care system are charging occupational therapy practitioners to provide evidence of the benefits of occupational therapy.

Check Your Thinking 6-1

Using your own words, describe occupation and occupation-based practice.

Compare your description with the descriptions in Chapter 1. Now ask your colleagues to describe occupation and occupation-based practice and compare your description with theirs. Consider the similarities and differences in the descriptions. Is there a right or wrong way of describing occupation and occupation-based practice? The purpose of this exercise is to demonstrate the variety of descriptions, each potentially acceptable, used by occupational therapy practitioners to describe occupation and occupation-based practice. As we discussed in Chapter 1, the literature presents a variety of definitions (Chisholm, Dolhi, & Schreiber, 2000; Clark, Azen, Zemke, et al., 1997; Pedretti & Early, 2001; Trombly, 2002) just as you and your colleagues may have different descriptions.

WHERE IS THE EVIDENCE: PROVE IT OR LOSE IT

How do occupational therapy practitioners prove that occupation-based practice facilitates a client's engagement in occupation that supports participation in a client's life? You may strongly believe that the interventions you include in your clients' occupational therapy programs are effective and improve your clients' occupational performance. You may also believe that the skilled services you provide positively impact the quality of life of your clients. Perhaps your clients would agree that occupational therapy was beneficial. Additionally, the interdisciplinary team may confirm that the inclusion of occupational therapy is a necessary service for their clients. But are your beliefs, your clients' agreement, and the team's confirmation enough? Does it prove that what we do and how we do it really works? Are subjective views considered evidence? And if so, is it enough evidence to validate the unique contribution of occupational therapy?

Simply put, it is *not* enough. The "move it or lose it" adage takes a different twist in the evidence-based practice arena of today's health care. For occupational therapy, and all health care professions, it becomes "prove it or lose it." The profession is at a pivotal point that has surpassed the information phase and moved into the evidence phase. So, how can you know that the intervention plan you design and implement with your clients enhances their occupational performance? The answer—you analyze and apply the existing evidence and/or generate additional evidence.

There has been a significant amount of theoretical support for occupation-based practice, but only modest pragmatic evidence to support the efficacy of occupation-based interventions. Nelson (1988) proposed that occupational therapy practitioners could, because of the belief that motivation is coupled to performance, use meaningful therapeutic adaptation to enhance client performance.

Additionally, Mary Reilly (1962) is often quoted—"Man, through the use of his hands, as they are energized by mind and will, can influence the state of his own health." Schmidt and Nelson (1996) reinforce Reilly's statement by emphasizing the positive relationship that exists between self-determined occupational participation and motivation.

We know that simply stating that something is a truth does not necessarily prove its truthfulness, nor does it provide the evidence that it is indeed a truth. Most people are cautious consumers when it comes to making a major purchase, such as a car or home. Would it not make sense that the consumers and payers of occupational therapy would use the same caution when purchasing our services? Although our historical literature advocates the use of occupation-based interventions, today's occupational therapy practitioners are charged with finding, reviewing, interpreting, using, and producing the evidence that can empirically support the use of occupation as intervention. Generating evidence that demonstrates the power of occupation to enhance participation in life has become essential for the profession.

REVIEWING THE LITERATURE

Finding and interpreting the existing literature is the first step in being an evidence-based practitioner. First, occupational therapy practitioners need to find relevant evidence that supports the interventions they use in practice. Next they need to read, interpret, and determine the applicability of the evidence to their clinical practice.

In order to conduct a comprehensive literature search you will need to utilize all available resources. The publications presented in this chapter were gathered by using several online databases including: OT SEARCH, Medline, Enterez-Pubmed, and the Cochran Database. In addition, publications were identified from reference lists and bibliographies from retrieved articles and hand-searches. The following keywords were used for the electronic searches: "occupation-based intervention," "occupation," "purposeful activity," and "added-purpose." This list of keywords for occupation-based intervention is not all-inclusive. Remember to explore terms associated with the keywords. When you include associated terms in your database search you may find relevant publications that would not be identified if you used only your original keyword(s).

Check Your Thinking 6-2

Refer to Step 1 of the practice analysis you completed in Chapter 4. What "client population" keywords would you use in combination with "occupation" keywords to search for literature relevant to your clinical practice?

OVERVIEW OF EVIDENCE

Table 6-1 is an overview of some of the evidence that addresses occupation-based practice. It is not intended to be a complete collection of evidence. New evidence is regularly being added to the literature, so routinely update and add to your list of articles related to your clinical question(s).

Table 6-1 presents the articles in chronological order by publication date and includes information as reported in the publication. Only the intervention category column represents our clinical interpretation. Any misrepresentation of information is unintentional. You are encouraged to obtain, review, and analyze the articles to determine their utility in your clinical practice. A table is included in Appendix E for you to use as you continue your exploration for literature related to occupation-based practice.

Table 6-1	An Overview of Evidence.

Intervention Category Key

A	=	Adjunctive intervention
E	=	Enabling intervention
P	=	Purposeful intervention
O	=	Occupation-based intervention

Note: The information in the purpose of study, population, and interventions columns is as it appears in the publication. The information in the intervention category column reflects our interpretation of the interventions based on the intervention continuum.

STUDY	PURPOSE OF STUDY	POPULATION	INTERVENTIONS	INTERVENTION CATEGORY
Kircher, 1984	To determine whether purposeful activity provides intrinsic motivation to exercise performance.	26 healthy adult females.	Jump rope activity.	P
			Jumping exercise without a rope.	E
Steinbeck, 1986	To examine if the presence of a purpose or a goal would have an effect on the number of times an individual would repeat a desired motion before reaching a point of perceived exertion.	30 healthy undergraduate students.	Purposeful lower extremity activity = woodworking activity (constructing a game) using a pedal-powered drill press.	P
			Nonpurposeful lower extremity activity = pedaling activity while depressing a lever.	E
			Purposeful upper extremity activity = playing a game (squeezing a rubber bulb to keep a Ping-Pong ball suspended in air).	P
			Nonpurposeful upper extremity activity = squeezing the rubber bulb (detached from the game).	E
Miller & Nelson, 1987	To examine the performance and affective meanings of individuals engaged in two different activities.	30 female undergraduate students.	Dual-purpose = stirring a substance for the purpose of exercise and making cookies.	P
			Exercise = stirring a substance for the purpose of exercise.	E
Mullins et al., 1987	To examine elderly nursing home residents' preference when presented with two kinds of exercise-type activity.	28 nursing home residents.	Exercise method II = stenciling a design located on a wall to make a wall hanging.	P
			Exercise method I = shoulder flexion exercise.	E

Table 6-1 An Overview of Evidence. *(continued)*

STUDY	PURPOSE OF STUDY	POPULATION	INTERVENTIONS	INTERVENTION CATEGORY
Thibodeaux & Ludwig, 1988	To investigate if purposeful activity is an intrinsic motivator.	15 healthy female college students.	Product-oriented activity = sanding a cutting board.	P
			Non-product-oriented activity = sanding a piece of wood.	E
Bloch et al., 1989 (Replication and extension of Kircher, 1984)	To determine whether purposeful activity provides intrinsic motivation to exercise.	30 healthy female college students.	Jump rope activity.	P
			Jumping exercise without a rope.	E
Yoder et al., 1989 (Extension of Miller & Nelson, 1987)	To examine performance of individuals in added-purpose, occupationally embedded exercise and rote exercise.	30 female nursing home residents.	Added-purpose, occupationally embedded exercise = stirring with materials and verbalizations synthesized to create an atmosphere of baking cookies.	P
			Rote exercise = stirring with no added environmental stimuli.	E
Licht & Nelson, 1990	To investigate the effects of an attempt to add meaning to a particular occupational situation.	30 nursing home residents.	Representational design copy task = line drawings representing objects familiar to the subjects (i.e., an arrow, a house, and a face).	E
			Nonrepresentational design copy task = line drawings of equal complexity but not representing objects.	E
Riccio et al., 1990	To examine the effects of verbally elicited imagery on movement.	27 female adult nursing home or foster care residents.	Rote-exercise = above head arm stretches and below waist arm stretches.	E
			Imagery-based = above head arm stretches as if picking apples and below waist arm stretches as if picking up coins.	E

(continues)

Table 6-1   An Overview of Evidence. *(continued)*

STUDY	PURPOSE OF STUDY	POPULATION	INTERVENTIONS	INTERVENTION CATEGORY
Bakshi et al., 1991	To examine the role of choice in purposeful and nonpurposeful activities.	20 healthy female students.	Purposeful activities = block printing with end product of wrapping paper; nail and thread art with end product of wall hanging; drill press with end product of Chinese checker board; rug hooking with end product of cushion cover; leather work with end product of book mark; weaving with end product of place mat; macrame with end product of plant hanger; and painting with end product of wrapping paper.	P
			Nonpurposeful activities = repetitive movements to simulate performance of block printing; nail and thread art; drill press; rug hooking; leather work; weaving; macramé; and painting but no end products.	E
Lang et al., 1992	To compare materials-based occupation, imagery-based occupation, and rote exercise.	18 nursing home residents.	Materials-based occupation = kicking a balloon.	E
			Imagery-based occupation = kicking foot while imagining kicking a balloon.	E
			Rote exercise = kicking foot.	E
Morton et al., 1992	To examine the effects of an added-purpose, task compared with a single-purpose task on performance.	30 employees of a health care facility.	Added-purpose task = ring a bell by moving a weight box along an angle frame.	E
			Single-purpose task = move a weight box along an angle frame.	E
DeKuiper et al., 1993 (Extension of Lang et al., 1992)	To explore the differences between a materials-based occupation, an imagery-based occupation, and rote exercise.	28 nursing home or retirement home residents.	Materials-based occupation = kicking a balloon.	E
			Imagery-based occupation = kicking foot while imagining kicking a balloon.	E
			Rote exercise = kicking foot.	E

Table 6-1   An Overview of Evidence. *(continued)*

STUDY	PURPOSE OF STUDY	POPULATION	INTERVENTIONS	INTERVENTION CATEGORY
King, 1993	To determine whether the use of a computer game as purposeful activity would increase the number of repetitions during grip and pinch strengthening activities.	146 hand therapy patients.	Purposeful activity = computer game operated by pinch and grip devices.	P
			Nonpurposeful activity = computer-directed exercise using pinch and grip devices.	E
Sietsema et al., 1993	To compare the movement elicited by occupationally embedded intervention with those elicited by rote exercise.	20 adults who had sustained traumatic brain injury.	Occupationally-embedded = play Simon™.	P
			Rote exercise = arm reach exercise.	E
Wu et al., 1994	To examine the effect of occupational form on reaching performance through kinematic analysis.	37 female college students.	Materials-based occupation = pick up a pencil from a pencil holder and prepare to write name.	P
			Imagery-based occupation = move arm while imagining picking up a pencil from a pencil holder and pretend to write name.	E
			Exercise = arm reach movement.	E
Yuen et al., 1994	To investigate the use of object-produced visual input in learning control of flexion and extension of an above-elbow training prosthesis.	52 healthy male college students.	Added-materials = use a flashlight attached to the hook of a prosthesis to connect dots on paper with light.	E
			Nonadded-materials = practice moving an equally weighted prosthesis without the light or dots.	E
Josephsson et al., 1995	To evaluate an intervention program aimed at supporting occupation.	4 older adults on a psychogeriatric day care unit.	One instrumental activity of daily living (i.e., prepare soft drink, brew and serve coffee, set table for coffee) was chosen for each subject based on observations and interviews with the subjects, their relatives, and staff.	O
Zimmerer-Branum & Nelson, 1995	To examine preferences between occupationally embedded exercise versus rote exercise.	52 nursing home residents.	Occupationally embedded exercise = unilateral dunking of a small, spongy ball into a basketball hoop.	P
			Rote exercise = arm movements simulating the dunking exercise.	E

(continues)

Table 6-1 An Overview of Evidence. *(continued)*

STUDY	PURPOSE OF STUDY	POPULATION	INTERVENTIONS	INTERVENTION CATEGORY
Hsieh et al., 1996	To investigate whether added-purpose occupations result in better performance than nonadded-purpose occupations.	21 adults with a diagnosis of unilateral cerebral hemiplegia.	Added-materials occupation = picking up and throwing a small ball with unimpaired hand.	E
			Imagery-based occupation = unimpaired arm movements while imagining picking up and throwing a small ball.	E
			Rote exercise = arm movements simulating picking up and throwing a small ball.	E
Nelson et al., 1996	To compare the effect of an occupationally embedded exercise with rote exercise.	28 adults post-cerebrovascular accident.	Occupationally embedded = arm exercise with a handle while playing a dice game.	P
			Rote exercise = arm exercise with a handle.	E
Schmidt & Nelson, 1996	To compare occupationally embedded exercise in an altruistic situation, occupationally embedded exercise that is not altruistic, and rote exercise.	19 adult inpatients who had an upper extremity strengthening component in their occupational therapy program.	Altruistic occupationally embedded exercise = sanding a board that would eventually become part of a rocking horse that would be given to the pediatric unit in the institution.	P
			Nonaltruistic occupationally embedded exercise = sanding a board that would eventually be made into a shelf for use somewhere in the institution.	P
			Rote exercise = sanding a board for exercise.	E
Thomas, 1996 (Extension of DeKuiper et al., 1993 and Lang et al., 1992)	To examine whether there is a difference among materials-based, imagery-based, and rote exercise occupational forms.	45 healthy females.	Materials-based occupation = kicking a balloon.	E
			Imagery-based occupation = kicking foot while imagining kicking a balloon.	E
			Rote exercise = kicking foot.	E

Table 6-1   An Overview of Evidence. *(continued)*

STUDY	PURPOSE OF STUDY	POPULATION	INTERVENTIONS	INTERVENTION CATEGORY
Clark et al., 1997	To evaluate the effectiveness of preventive occupational therapy services.	361 independent older adults.	Occupational therapy = modular programmatic units centered on topics such as home and community safety, transportation utilization, joint protection, adaptive equipment, energy conservation, exercise, and nutrition. Included self-analysis.	O
			Social activity = activities designed to encourage social interaction among members such as community outings, craft projects, viewing films, playing games, and attending dances.	P
			Nontreatment = no intervention.	Not applicable
Dean & Shepherd, 1997	To evaluate the effect of a 2-week task-related training program.	20 adults post-stroke at least 12 months with resulting hemiplegia.	Task-related training = reaching tasks beyond arm's length designed to improve balance.	E
			Sham training = manipulative tasks within arm's length.	E
Ferguson & Trombly, 1997	To examine the effects of both added-purpose and meaningful occupation on motor learning.	20 college students.	Added-purpose exercise = practice note patterns using an electric keyboard to produce a musical tune.	P
			Rote exercise = practice note patterns using an electric keyboard without tune production.	E
Lin et al., 1997	Meta-analysis focusing on the relationship between occupational form and occupational performance.	17 studies.	Not applicable.	Not applicable
Kellegrew, 1998	To explore the relationship between opportunities for occupation and skill performance.	3 caregivers of children with disabilities.	Creating occupation opportunities = caregiver education (information focusing on targeted self-care occupations), and caregiver performance of targeted self-care intervention with child.	O
			Typical routine = no intervention.	Not applicable

(continues)

Table 6-1   An Overview of Evidence. *(continued)*

STUDY	PURPOSE OF STUDY	POPULATION	INTERVENTIONS	INTERVENTION CATEGORY
Sakemiller & Nelson, 1998	To examine whether play elicits therapeutic patterns of movement.	2 female children with hypotonic cerebral palsy.	Play embedded exercise = facilitation of vertical neck and back extension with performance of subject-identified favorite game.	O
			Nonplay embedded exercise = facilitation of vertical neck and back extension without performance of game.	E
Christiansen et al., 1999	To explore the relationship between occupation and subjective well-being.	120 adults.	No intervention = exploratory study collected data on characteristics of occupation, subjective well-being, personality type, and demographics through self-administered questionnaires.	Not applicable
Rebeiro & Cook, 1999	To investigate the occupation-as-means experience.	8 members of an outpatient, women's mental health group.	Occupation of choice (for the group) = making a quilt.	O
Thomas et al., 1999	To investigate whether patients undergoing Phase II cardiac rehabilitation perform differently during materials-based, imagery-based, and rote exercise-based occupational forms.	15 outpatients undergoing Phase II cardiac rehabilitation.	Materials-based = hip abduction movement while performing a ball-kicking game.	P
			Imagery-based = hip abduction movement while imagining performance of a ball-kicking game.	E
			Rote exercise-based = hip abduction movement.	E
Hartman et al., 2000	To explore whether children engaged in hands-on learning of an occupation would have better recall than children engaged in a demonstration teaching method.	73 healthy third graders.	Hands-on = made a model of a volcano.	P
			Demonstration = observed someone making a model of a volcano.	A
Holm et al., 2000	To examine the effect of three occupations-based interventions for reducing the frequency of dysfunctional behaviors.	2 female residents of a Community Living Arrangement.	Occupations at school and sheltered workshop = everyday occupations in conjunction with behavior modification program.	O
			Morning occupations = focused on participation in routine morning occupations versus dysfunctional behaviors with a positive reinforcement for participation.	O

| **Table 6-1** | An Overview of Evidence. *(continued)* | | | |

STUDY	PURPOSE OF STUDY	POPULATION	INTERVENTIONS	INTERVENTION CATEGORY
Holm et al., *(continued)*			Evening occupations = focused on participation in routine afternoon and evening occupations, including leisure activities with positive reinforcement for participation.	O
Melchert-McKearnan et al., 2000	To compare measures of pain when children with burn injuries were engaged in a purposeful play activity versus rote exercise.	2 male children.	Purposeful play activity = repetitions of movements within a set range-of-motion goal while playing a game that was identified by the child as an activity that he enjoyed doing.	O
			Rote exercise = repetitions of movements within a set range-of-motion goal.	E
Ross & Nelson, 2000 (Replication and extension of Wu et al., 1994)	To examine the effect of occupational form on reaching performance through kinematic analysis.	60 healthy female college students.	Materials-based occupation = pick up a pencil from a pencil holder and prepare to write name.	P
			Imagery-based occupation = move arm while imagining picking up a pencil from a pencil holder and pretend to write name.	E
			Exercise = arm reach movement.	E
Venable et al., 2000	To clarify the relationship between the occupation of exercise, functional ability, and volition.	48 community dwelling adults.	Social/craft activities = e.g., ceramics, Grandmother's Club, Bridge Club, quilting, and a Senior Luncheon/Lecture series.	O
			Social/craft activities plus exercise = social/craft activities plus individual exercise.	O
			Exercise/dance = exercise or dance class.	O
Clark et al., 2001 (Follow-up of Clark et al., 1997)	To explore the long-term health effects of preventive occupational therapy.	285 independent older adults.	Occupational therapy = modular programmatic units centered on topics such as home and community safety, transportation utilization, joint protection, adaptive equipment, energy conservation, exercise, and nutrition. Included self-analysis.	O

(continues)

| Table 6-1 | An Overview of Evidence. *(continued)* |

STUDY	PURPOSE OF STUDY	POPULATION	INTERVENTIONS	INTERVENTION CATEGORY
Clark et al., *(continued)*			Social activity = activities designed to encourage social interaction among members such as community outings, craft projects, viewing films, playing games, and attending dances.	P
			Nontreatment = no intervention.	Not applicable
Eakman & Nelson, 2001	To explore the use of "active occupations."	30 males with closed head injuries.	Hands-on = verbal instruction and manipulation of the utensils and ingredients for making meatballs.	P
			Verbal training only = verbal instruction and reading the steps of making meatballs.	E
Jackson & Schkade, 2001	To compare the effectiveness of the Occupational Adaptation frame of reference with the biomechanical-rehabilitation model.	40 older adults post-hip fracture.	Occupational Adaptation Model = client choice of all tasks; client able to control therapy process by working on tasks important to client.	O
			Biomechanical-Rehabilitation Model = exercises and activities of the facility protocol.	E & P
Nagel & Rice, 2001	To investigate cross-transfer effects during an occupationally embedded task that involved learning a fine motor skill.	48 healthy undergraduate and graduate students.	Training = training to perform toy maze, an instruction sheet, and verbal instruction; requested to complete the toy maze three times a day for seven days using left hand.	P
			No-training = no materials or instruction.	Not applicable
Tham et al., 2001	To evaluate the effect of an intervention program focused on improving the awareness of disabilities.	4 female adult right brain damage.	Disability awareness = occupational inpatients with therapy focused on training awareness of disability plus "traditional."	O
			Traditional = occupational therapy focused on training in self-care activities by using the participant's available abilities and by adapting task demands and contexts.	P

				INTERVENTION
STUDY	PURPOSE OF STUDY	POPULATION	INTERVENTIONS	CATEGORY
Fasoli et al., 2002	To explore whether materials-based occupation elicited better movement organization than imagery-based occupation.	5 adults with left brain damage following cerebrovasular accident and 5 adults without history of neurological impairment.	Materials-based = tools and objects available for task completion. Imagery-based = pretend to perform an action with no tool, or no object of the tool's action present.	P E

Table 6-1   An Overview of Evidence. *(continued)*

BECOMING AN EVIDENCE-BASED PRACTITIONER: HOW CAN I GET STARTED?

Does the word "research" scare you? If so, you are not alone. Participating in research does not necessarily involve jumping in headfirst or starting from scratch. You can (and should) start with activities that will increase your comfort level with research. With the right experience and mentor, your motivation and investment in finding, reviewing, interpreting, using, and even producing evidence can be heightened. The following ideas can help get you started on the road to becoming an evidence-based practitioner.

1. Start a journal club to review current literature.

   Suggestions for starting a journal club:

   > A good size for a journal club is four to eight members.

   > Each meeting should focus on one article and have one person leading the discussion.

   > Choose an article that relates to your client population.

   > Each participant should read the article prior to the group meeting.

   > Consider discussing the following questions:

   >> What is the research question the study is trying to answer?

   >> What are the hypotheses?

   >> What is the study design?

   >> Who were the subjects?

   >> What is being measured?

What are the tools or instruments used to measure the target outcomes?

What are the results?

How do the authors interpret their findings?

Could you replicate the study based on the information in the article?

What are the strengths and limitations of the study?

What could the researchers have done to make the study better?

How can the results be applied in your clinical practice?

2. If you don't have the time to meet face-to-face in a formal journal club, consider establishing an online journal club.

3. Identify research questions applicable to your practice setting and client population based on your journal club discussions.

4. Maintain an ongoing list of potential clinical questions that you and your colleagues want to answer. Questions may focus on a particular condition, occupational performance deficit, or the effectiveness of a particular occupational therapy intervention. Keep the list visible in your office for easy access. Now, brainstorm and list possible strategies to answer your clinical questions.

Interpreting evidence can be an overwhelming task. The key to interpretation is reading and discussing. It is important to understand that the process of reading and discussing an article will need to be repeated in order for you and your colleagues to adequately understand the study, its findings, and its application to your clinical practice. The more you do it—read and discuss—the easier it becomes. Seek out evidence-learning opportunities through your local educational institutions. Seek out evidence mentors. Practitioners who are actively engaged in research are usually eager to share their expertise with an interested practitioner. As you pursue these opportunities, don't forget to ask how you can become involved in generating evidence.

Whether you realize it or not, you are already engaging in the research process and generating evidence. As an occupational therapy practitioner, you collect data on a daily basis. Your documentation related to client status, progress, and goal attainment is a source of data. For example, your client's ability to more safely and/or independently prepare a meal at discharge compared to performance on admission can help support the efficacy of the interventions you have included in your client's occupational therapy intervention plan. As you engage in the occupational therapy process you are identifying clinical questions; establishing hypotheses; identifying outcomes; designing services; collecting, analyzing, and interpreting data; and reporting findings—all of which parallel the steps of the research process.

Summary

The intent of this chapter has been two-fold. First, we hope we have heightened your awareness of the need to use and contribute to the evidence that supports the use of occupation-based interventions. Second, by including some of the literature related to occupation-based practice, we have provided you with a starting point. We encourage you to identify the evidence that relates to your clinical practice, critically read and analyze the evidence, determine its application to your clinical practice, and use it. But don't stop with the publications identified in this chapter. Keep going—identify, gather, read, analyze, discuss, and apply the evidence to your clinical practice.

References

Bakshi, R., Bhambhani, Y., & Madill, H. (1991). The effects of task preference on performance during purposeful and nonpurposeful activities. *American Journal of Occupational Therapy, 45,* 912–916.

Bloch, M. W., Smith, D. A., & Nelson, D. L. (1989). Heart rate, activity, duration, and affect in added-purpose versus single-purpose jumping activities. *American Journal of Occupational Therapy, 43,* 25–30.

Bury, T. J., & Mead, J. M. (1998). *Evidence-based healthcare: A practical guide for therapists.* Oxford, England: Butterworth-Heinemann.

Chisholm, D., Dolhi, C., & Schreiber, J. (2000). Creating occupation-based opportunities in a medical model clinical practice setting. *OT Practice, 5* (1), CE1–8.

Christiansen, C. H., Backman, C., Little, B. R., & Nguyen, A. (1999). Occupational and well-being: A study of personal projects. *American Journal of Occupational Therapy, 53,* 91–100.

Clark, F., Azen, S. P., Carlson, M., Mandel, D., LeBree, L., Hay, J., et al. (2001). Embedding health-promoting changes into the daily lives of independent-living older adults: Long-term follow-up of occupational therapy intervention. *Journal of Gerontology, 56B,* P60–P63.

Clark, F., Azen, S. P., Zemke, R., Jackson, J., Carlson, M., Mandel, D., et al. (1997). Occupational therapy for independent-living older adults: A randomized controlled trial. *Journal of the American Medical Association, 278,* 1321–1326.

Dean, C. M., & Shepherd, R. B. (1997). Task-related training improves performance of seated reaching tasks after stroke: A randomized controlled trial. *Stroke, 28,* 722–728.

DeKuiper, W. P., Nelson, D. L., & White, B. E. (1993). Materials-based occupation versus imagery-based occupation versus rote exercise: A replication and extension. *Occupational Therapy Journal of Research, 13,* 183–197.

Eakman, A. M., & Nelson, D. L. (2001). The effects of hands-on occupation on recall memory in men with traumatic brain injuries. *Occupational Therapy Journal of Research, 21,* 109–114.

Fasoli, S. E., Trombly, C. A., Tickle-Degnen, L., & Verfaellie, M. H. (2002). Context and goal-directed movement: The effect of materials-based occupation. *Occupational Therapy Journal of Research, 22,* 119–128.

Ferguson, J. M., & Trombly, C. A. (1997). The effect of added-purpose and meaningful occupation on motor learning. *American Journal of Occupational Therapy, 51*, 508–515.

Hartman, B. A., Miller, B. K., & Nelson, D. L. (2000). The effects of hands-on occupation versus demonstration on children's recall memory. *American Journal of Occupational Therapy, 54*, 477–483.

Holm, M. B., Santangelo, M. A., Fromuth, D. J., Brown, S. O., & Walter, H. (2000). Effectiveness of everyday occupations for changing client behaviors in a community living arrangement. *American Journal of Occupational Therapy, 54*, 361–371.

Hsieh, C., Nelson, D. L., Smith, D. A., & Peterson, C. Q. (1996). A comparison of performance in added-purpose occupations and rote exercise for dynamic standing balance in persons with hemiplegia. *American Journal of Occupational Therapy, 50*, 10–16.

Jackson, J. P., & Schkade, J. K. (2001). Occupation Adaptation model versus biomechanical-rehabilitation model in the treatment of patients with hip fractures. *American Journal of Occupational Therapy, 55*, 531–537.

Josephsson, S., Backman, L., Borell, L., Nygard, L., & Bernspang, B. (1995). Effectiveness of an intervention to improve occupational performance in dementia. *Occupational Therapy Journal of Research, 15*, 36–49.

Kellegrew, D. H. (1998). Creating opportunities for occupation: An intervention to promote the self-care independence of young children with special needs. *American Journal of Occupational Therapy, 52*, 457–465.

King, T. I. (1993). Hand strengthening with a computer for purposeful activity. *American Journal of Occupational Therapy, 47*, 635–637.

Kircher, M. A. (1984). Motivation as a factor of perceived exertion in purposeful versus non-purposeful activity. *American Journal of Occupational Therapy, 38*, 165–170.

Lang, E. M., Nelson, D. L., & Bush, M. A. (1992). Comparison of performance in materials-based occupation, imagery-based occupation, and rote exercise in nursing home residents. *American Journal of Occupational Therapy, 46*, 607–611.

Law, M. (2002). *Evidence-based rehabilitation: A guide to practice.* Thorofare, NJ: Slack, Inc.

Licht, B. C., & Nelson, D. L. (1990). Adding meaning to a design copy task through representational stimuli. *American Journal of Occupational Therapy, 44*, 408–413.

Lin, K., Wu, C., Tickle-Degnen, L., & Coster, W. (1997). Enhancing occupational performance through occupationally embedded exercise: A meta-analytic review. *Occupational Therapy Journal of Research, 17*, 25–47.

Melchert-McKearnan, K., Deitz, J., Engel, J. M., & White, O. (2000). Children with burn injuries: Purposeful activity versus rote exercise. *American Journal of Occupational Therapy, 54*, 381–390.

Miller, L., & Nelson, D. L. (1987). Dual-purpose activity versus single-purpose activity in terms of duration of task, exertion level, and affect. *Occupational Therapy in Mental Health, 7*, 55–67.

Morton, G. G., Barnett, D. W., & Hale, L. S. (1992). A comparison of performance measures of an added-purpose task versus a single-purpose task for upper extremities. *American Journal of Occupational Therapy, 46*, 128–133.

Mullins, C. S., Nelson, D. L., & Smith, D. A. (1987). Exercise through dual-purpose activity in the institutionalized elderly. *Physical and Occupational Therapy in Geriatrics, 5*(3), 29–39.

Nagel, M. J., & Rice, M. S. (2001). Cross transfer effects in the upper extremity during an occupationally embedded exercise. *American Journal of Occupational Therapy, 55,* 317–323.

Nelson, D. L. (1988). Occupation: Form and performance. *American Journal of Occupational Therapy, 42,* 633–641.

Nelson, D. L., Konosky, K., Fleharty, K., Webb, R., Newer, K., Hazboun, V. P., et al. (1996). The effects of an occupationally embedded exercise on bilaterally assisted supination in persons with hemiplegia. *American Journal of Occupational Therapy, 50,* 639–646.

Pedretti, L. W., & Early, M. B. (2001). Occupational performance: A model for practice in physical dysfunction. In L. W. Pedretti & M. B. Early (Eds.), *Occupational therapy: Practice skills for physical dysfunction* (5th ed., pp. 7–9). St. Louis: Mosby.

Portney, L. G., & Watkins, M. P. (2000). *Foundations of clinical research: Applications to practice* (2nd ed.). Upper Saddle River, NJ: Prentice-Hall, Inc.

Rebeiro, K. L., & Cook, J. V. (1999). Opportunity, not prescription: An exploratory study of the experience of occupational engagement. *Canadian Journal of Occupational Therapy, 66,* 176–187.

Reilly, M. (1962). Occupational therapy can be one of the great ideas of 20th century medicine. *American Journal of Occupational Therapy, 25,* 243–246.

Riccio, C. M., Nelson, D. L., & Bush, M. A. (1990). Adding purpose to the repetitive exercise of elderly women through imagery. *American Journal of Occupational Therapy, 44,* 714–719.

Ross, L. M., & Nelson, D. L. (2000). Comparing materials-based occupation, imagery-based occupation, and rote movement through kinematic analysis of reach. *Occupational Therapy Journal of Research, 20,* 45–60.

Sackett, D. L., Straus, S. E., Richardson, W. S., Rosenberg, W., & Haynes, R. B. (2000). *Evidence-based medicine: How to practice and teach EBM.* Edinburgh, Scotland: Churchill Livingstone.

Sakemiller, L. M., & Nelson, D. L. (1998). Eliciting functional extension in prone through the use of a game [case report]. *American Journal of Occupational Therapy, 52,* 150–157.

Schmidt, C. L., & Nelson, D. L. (1996). A comparison of three occupation forms in rehabilitation patients receiving upper extremity strengthening. *Occupational Therapy Journal of Research, 16,* 200–215.

Sietsema, J. M., Nelson, D. L., Mulder, R. M., Mervau-Scheidel, D., & White, B. E. (1993). The use of a game to promote arm reach in persons with traumatic brain injury. *American Journal of Occupational Therapy, 47,* 19–24.

Steinbeck, T. M. (1986). Purposeful activity and performance. *American Journal of Occupational Therapy, 40,* 529–534.

Tham, K., Ginsburg, E., Fisher, A. G., & Tegner, R. (2001). Training to improve awareness of disabilities in clients with unilateral neglect. *American Journal of Occupational Therapy, 55,* 46–54.

Thibodeaux, C. S., & Ludwig, F. M. (1988). Intrinsic motivation in product-oriented and non-product-oriented activities. *American Journal of Occupational Therapy, 42,* 169–175.

Thomas, J. J. (1996). Materials-based, imagery-based, and rote exercise occupational forms: Effect on repetitions, heart rate, duration of performance, and self-perceived rest period in well elderly women. *American Journal of Occupational Therapy, 50,* 783–789.

Thomas, J. J., Wyk, S. V., & Boyer, J. (1999). Contrasting occupational forms: Effects on performance and affect in patients undergoing Phase II cardiac rehabilitation. *Occupational Therapy Journal of Research, 19,* 187–202.

Trombly, C. A. (2002). Occupation. In C. A. Trombly & M. V. Randomski (Eds.), *Occupational therapy for physical dysfunction* (5th ed., pp. 255–281). Philadelphia: Lippincott, Williams & Wilkins.

Venable, E., Hanson, D., Shechtman, O., & Dasler, P. (2000). The effects of exercise on occupational functioning in the well elderly. *Physical and Occupational Therapy in Geriatrics, 17,* 29–42.

Wu, C., Trombly, C. A., & Lin, K. (1994). The relationship between occupational form and occupational performance: A kinematic perspective. *American Journal of Occupational Therapy, 48,* 679–687.

Yoder, R. M., Nelson, D. L., & Smith, D. A. (1989). Added-purpose versus rote exercise in female nursing home residents. *American Journal of Occupational Therapy, 43,* 581–586.

Yuen, H. K., Nelson, D. L., Peterson, C. Q., & Dickinson, A. (1994). Prosthesis training as a context for studying occupational forms and motoric adaptation. *American Journal of Occupational Therapy, 48,* 55–61.

Zimmerer-Branum, S., & Nelson, D. L. (1995). Occupationally embedded exercise versus rote exercise: A choice between occupational forms by elderly nursing home residents. *American Journal of Occupational Therapy, 49,* 397–402.

Suggested Readings

In addition to the references listed in this chapter, the following are useful information sources for evidence-based practice.

Bhavnani, G. (2000, December). Toward occupation-based practice in hand rehabilitation. *Physical Disabilities—Special Interest Section Quarterly, 23,* 1–2.

Karas, M. A., & Daly, J. J. (1997). *Clinical research and documentation: Single-subject research designs and documentation for the neurologically impaired adult.* Chicago, IL: Neurodevelopmental Treatment Association, Inc.

Laliberte-Rudman, D., Yu, B., Scott, E., & Pajouhandeh, P. (2000). Exploration of the perspectives of persons with schizophrenia regarding quality of life. *American Journal of Occupational Therapy, 54,* 137–147.

Rebeiro, K. L. (2000). Client perspectives on occupational therapy practice: Are we truly client-centered? *Canadian Journal of Occupational Therapy, 67,* 7–14.

Rebeiro, K. L. (2001). Enabling occupation: The importance of an affirming environment. *Canadian Journal of Occupational Therapy, 68,* 80–89.

Royeen, C. B. (1997). *A research primer in occupational and physical therapy.* Bethesda, MD: American Occupational Therapy Association, Inc.

Unruh, A. M., Smith, N., & Scammell, C. (2000). The occupation of gardening in life threatening illness: A qualitative pilot project. *Canadian Journal of Occupational Therapy, 67,* 70–77.

Clinical Scenarios

Learning Objectives

After reading this chapter and completing the learning activities, you should be able to do the following:

1. Identify problems and strengths for a client based on the occupational profile and analysis of occupational performance information.
2. Identify areas of occupation, performance skills, performance patterns, and/or performance contexts to address in a client's occupational therapy intervention plan.
3. Identify interventions for a client using the occupational profile and analysis of occupational performance information, identified strengths and problems, and results of a client-centered interview.
4. Categorize interventions in a client's occupational therapy intervention plan within the intervention continuum.
5. Develop plans for an occupational therapy session for a client that facilitates movement toward occupation-based intervention.
6. Consider and respond to potential clinical reasoning dilemmas.

INTRODUCTION

This chapter is designed to provide you with the opportunity to develop occupational therapy intervention plans using the intervention continuum as a tool for clinical reasoning. This process will assist you in improving your clinical reasoning skills so that the inclusion of occupation-based interventions becomes part of your clinical habit pattern. The clinical scenarios provided in this chapter (Table 7-1) were created to include a variety of practice settings and client populations. The information provided in the scenarios is fictitious. We have purposely provided only general information and limited details, as you are encouraged to add, change, or delete information in order to enhance or refocus the clinical scenario to fit your practice setting, client population, and knowledge base.

The format for the clinical scenarios is outlined in Table 7-2. The sample interventions and session plans provided in this chapter are not intended to reflect best practice nor any treatment protocol, but are included solely to provide guidance for the development of interventions for each case. The information provided in the

Table 7-1			Overview of Clinical Scenarios.	
NAME	**GENDER**	**AGE**	**PRIMARY DIAGNOSIS**	**PRACTICE SETTING**
Allison	female	17	Acquired brain injury	Inpatient rehabilitation facility
Becca	female	52	Hip replacement	Acute care hospital
Charles	male	76	Parkinson's disease	Skilled nursing facility
Dave	male	68	Dementia	Acute care hospital
George	male	63	End stage cardiac disease	Home hospice
Jean	female	82	Chronic obstructive pulmonary disease	Long-term care facility
Kay	female	66	Cerebrovascular accident	Assisted living facility
Maura	female	8	Learning disability and attention deficit/hyperactivity disorder	School classroom
Miguel	male	20	C5 tetraplegia, complete	Inpatient rehabilitation facility
Pam	female	42	Carpal tunnel syndrome	Outpatient hand clinic
Stephen	male	3	Down's syndrome	Preschool
Terrell	male	60	C4–6 disketomy	Home care
Trudy	female	31	Substance abuse	Community drop-in center
Walter	male	28	Schizophrenia	Acute care hospital

Table 7-2	Clinical Scenarios Format.
Occupational Profile and Analysis of Occupational Performance	Provides a general description of the client's premorbid functional level, home, and social environments. Limited information related to the client's current occupational performance is offered.
Identification of Strengths and Problems	Based on the occupational profile and analysis of occupational performance, you identify the client's strengths and problem areas.
Identification of Areas of Occupation, Performance Skills, Performance Patterns, and Performance Contexts	You make a list of the areas of occupation, performance skills, performance patterns, and/or performance contexts (refer to Appendix F) that you anticipate addressing in the client's occupational therapy intervention plan.
Client-Centered Interview Results	Provides you with a list of the occupations that the client identified as needing, wanting, and being expected to perform and with the client's priority areas for improvement.
Intervention Brainstorm	Based on the client's occupational profile and analysis of occupational performance, the strengths and problems, and the client-centered interview, you brainstorm a list of potential interventions that you anticipate including in the client's occupational therapy intervention plan.
Intervention Continuum	You categorize each of the interventions that you developed in the Intervention Brainstorm according to the intervention continuum.
Sample Intervention Continuum	Provides you with sample interventions for the client categorized in the intervention continuum.
Session Plan—Intervention Continuum	You develop two sample treatment sessions using the interventions that you generated in the Intervention Brainstorm.
Sample Session Plans	Two sample sessions are provided that incorporate the interventions provided in the Sample Intervention Continuum.
Check Your Thinking	You identify the client's priority occupations that have been addressed in the sample session plans.
What If	You consider a variety of situations to challenge your clinical reasoning skills related to the clinical scenario.

clinical scenarios is for the purpose of assisting you in understanding how the concept of occupation-based practice can be integrated into a variety of clinical situations. The interventions described in the clinical scenarios are *not* to be used as practice guidelines for providing occupational therapy services for your "real life" clients. You, the occupational therapy practitioner, are responsible for using clinical judgment regarding the appropriateness of any given intervention as determined by an individual's unique circumstances.

Appendix G includes a blank clinical scenario form. This form is provided so that you can use it in your clinical practice to assist you in integrating occupation-based interventions into your clients' intervention plans.

CLINICAL SCENARIO #1—ALLISON

Setting:	Inpatient rehabilitation facility
Diagnosis:	Acquired brain injury
Estimated duration of intervention:	Two to three weeks
Anticipated discharge plan:	Home with family; return to school

Occupational Profile and Analysis of Occupational Performance

Allison is a 17-year-old high school senior. She sustained a closed head injury as a result of a motor vehicle accident. Prior to her injury, Allison lived at home with her parents and was involved in school and extracurricular activities, including college preparatory classes, playing for her high school softball team, and actively participating in the debate club, drama club, and her church youth group. Once a week, Allison volunteered at a homeless shelter, where she prepared and served meals to needy members of her local community. Her family is very supportive and actively involved in her recovery; however, they have little experience with the health care system and limited knowledge of Allison's condition.

Allison is pleasant, cooperative, and is oriented to person, place, and time. She appears slightly lethargic but is easily aroused. No motor impairments are noted, but she reports decreased endurance and frequent headaches. Based on standardized testing, Allison displays some memory and cognitive deficits with severe impairment in the areas of visual memory and sequencing, multiple digit math skills, and concrete problem solving/mental flexibility. Despite visual acuity being within functional limits, Allison reports visual fatigue, pain described as "eye strain," and difficulty focusing her eyes. She is unable to read for more than a few minutes at a time and has difficulty concentrating and organizing the information she reads.

Identification of Strengths and Problems

Make a list of Allison's strengths and problems based on your review of her occupational profile and analysis of occupational performance.

My List of Allison's Strengths:

My List of Allison's Problems:

Identification of Areas of Occupation, Performance Skills, Performance Patterns, and Performance Contexts

Using Appendix F, make a list of the areas of occupation, performance skills, performance patterns, and/or performance contexts that you anticipate addressing in Allison's occupational therapy intervention plan.

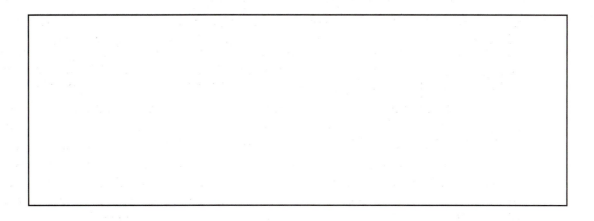

Client-Centered Interview Results

The following is Allison's client-centered interview, which includes a list of the occupations she identified as needing, wanting, and being expected to perform. The occupations Allison identified as priority areas for improvement are circled.

Occupations I need to do:

(1.) Go to school

2. Take a shower every morning

3. Sleep

4. Get dressed

(5.) Go shopping with my friends

Occupations I want to do:

(1.) Volunteer at the shelter

2. Be in my school play

(3.) Be with my friends—chat online and go to the mall

4. Play softball

5. Go to my church youth group

Occupations I am expected to do:

1. Make my bed

2. Help with dinner

3. Catch the bus on time

4. Walk the dog

(5.) Do my homework

Intervention Brainstorm

Make a list of interventions to include in Allison's occupational therapy intervention plan based on Allison's occupational profile and analysis of occupational performance, the strengths and problems you identified, and Allison's client-centered interview results.

Intervention Continuum

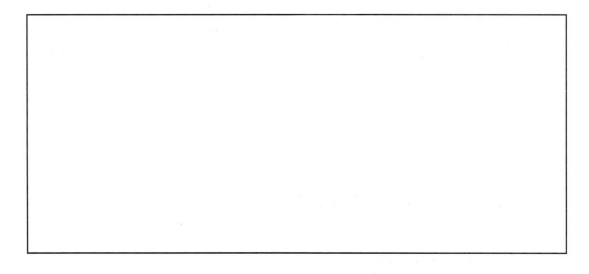

Adjunctive	**Enabling**	**Purposeful**	**Occupation-Based**
Interventions that prepare for performance and participation	*Interventions that focus on performance skills*	*Interventions that have a pre-determined goal and facilitate practice and problem solving*	*Interventions that are perceived as desirable, match individualized goals, and occur in appropriate context*

The next step is to categorize the interventions you identified in the Intervention Brainstorm activity according to the intervention continuum. Designate the category into which each intervention falls by labeling the interventions as "A," "E," "P," or "O" to reflect them as adjunctive, enabling, purposeful, or occupation-based.

Sample Intervention Continuum

Sample interventions categorized in the intervention continuum that may be included in Allison's occupational therapy intervention plan follow.

A Adjunctive Interventions	**E** Enabling Interventions	**P** Purposeful Interventions	**O** Occupation-Based Interventions
Provide a logbook and calculator for compensation with memory and math applications. *Provide an alarm clock watch for short-term memory and time management.* *Provide family with literature pertaining to brain injury and available support services.*	*Complete worksheets and flashcards to relearn and practice fundamental math operations.* *Read words of various sized fonts and determine the best size font to be used for written materials.*	*Apply math skills by calculating prices from store advertisements.* *Make purchases in the hospital cafeteria or gift shop.* *Bake cookies in the occupational therapy clinic kitchen.* *Play a card game requiring simple math problem-solving skills.*	*Go to the mall on a community outing and make purchases with own money.* *Plan a "typical day" in anticipation of discharge in order to maintain a structured daily routine.* *Organize and prepare lunch for herself and two of her friends in the clinic kitchen.*

Session Plan—Intervention Continuum

Identify one of Allison's priority occupations:

Using interventions from the "Intervention Brainstorm," develop an occupational therapy session for Allison.

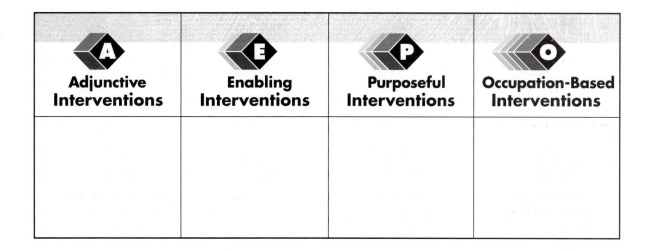

Adjunctive Interventions	Enabling Interventions	Purposeful Interventions	Occupation-Based Interventions

Now develop a second occupational therapy session for Allison. Consider progressing to the next session or to a session that is closer to the discontinuation of occupational therapy services.

Identify which of Allison's priority occupation(s) will be addressed in this session:

Adjunctive Interventions	Enabling Interventions	Purposeful Interventions	Occupation-Based Interventions

Sample Session Plans

Two sample session plans that may be included in Allison's occupational therapy intervention follow.

Session Plan #1

A Adjunctive Interventions	**E** Enabling Interventions	**P** Purposeful Interventions	**O** Occupation-Based Interventions
Provide a logbook and calculator for compensation with memory and math applications.	*Allison completes worksheets and flashcards to relearn and practice fundamental math operations.*	*Allison applies math skills by calculating prices from store advertisements.* *Allison makes purchases in the hospital gift shop.*	

Session Plan #2

A Adjunctive Interventions	**E** Enabling Interventions	**P** Purposeful Interventions	**O** Occupation-Based Interventions
			Allison goes to the mall on a community outing where she can make purchases with her own money.

Check Your Thinking 7-1

Review the sample sessions and Allison's client-centered interview. Which of Allison's priority occupations do you think each sample session addressed?

Session #1:

Session #2:

What If?

Consider how each of the following "what if?" situations would affect your intervention plan for Allison.

1. What if Allison has physical impairments in addition to her cognitive impairments, such as left-sided weakness, which require her to use a walker and receive close supervision during ambulation?

2. What if Allison exhibits additional cognitive deficits including impulsivity, poor judgment, or safety awareness?

3. What if Allison is a depressed teenager who is disinterested in school, peers, and her family and only wants to go home?

4. What if Allison is a single mother and is responsible for the care of her 2-year-old daughter?

CLINICAL SCENARIO #2—BECCA

Setting:	Acute care hospital
Diagnoses:	Status-post right hip replacement; degenerative joint disease; Type I diabetes
Estimated duration of intervention:	Three days
Anticipated discharge plan:	Reside temporarily with son and daughter-in-law

Occupational Profile and Analysis of Occupational Performance

Becca is a 52-year-old female who lives with her husband in a two-story home with 15 steps to enter. Her bedroom and bathroom are located on the second floor and laundry facilities are in the basement. Prior to this surgery, she was a full-time homemaker and was independent in all self-care tasks, meal preparation, light home management, and financial management. Becca's son and daughter-in-law and their four children reside approximately 30 miles from her home. She attends all of her grandchildren's sporting and school events. She was socially active prior to her surgery including singing regularly in her church choir and being the chairperson of the monthly fellowship dinner committee. Becca does not drive and uses public transportation. Her husband's job requires weekly travel, and he is away from home for four to five days each week.

Becca is pleasant and cooperative. She exhibits no deficits in cognition, vision, or hearing; however, she describes symptoms consistent with the initial onset of peripheral neuropathy. Upper extremity functioning is within normal limits for range of motion and coordination. She exhibits fair + (3+) proximal upper extremity strength during manual muscle testing. Distal upper extremity strength is within functional limits. She requires moderate assistance for bed mobility and bed-to-wheelchair transfers with frequent cues to adhere to hip precautions and weight-bearing-as-tolerated status. She reports some pain in her hip during movement and expresses a fear of "popping her hip out." Becca reports feeling anxious in anticipation of attending therapy.

Identification of Strengths and Problems

Make a list of Becca's strengths and problems based on your review of her occupational profile and analysis of occupational performance.

> **My List of Becca's Strengths:**

My List of Becca's Problems:

Identification of Areas of Occupation, Performance Skills, Performance Patterns, and Performance Contexts

Using Appendix F, make a list of the areas of occupation, performance skills, performance patterns, and/or performance contexts that you anticipate addressing in Becca's occupational therapy intervention plan.

Client-Centered Interview Results

The following is Becca's client-centered interview, which includes a list of the occupations that she identified as needing, wanting, and being expected to perform. The occupations Becca identified as priority areas for improvement are circled.

Occupations I need to do:

1. Go grocery shopping

2. Get bathed and dressed

3. Prepare my meals

4. Clean my home

5. Go to church

Occupations I want to do:

①. Visit with my grandchildren

②. Take the bus

3. Maintain my garden

4. Clean my home

5. Go to church

Occupations I am expected to do:

1. Go to choir practice

2. Pay my bills

3. Help with church dinners

4. Visit my grandchildren

⑤. Clean my home

Intervention Brainstorm

Make a list of interventions to include in Becca's occupational therapy intervention plan based on Becca's occupational profile and analysis of occupational performance, the strengths and problems you identified, and Becca's client-centered interview results.

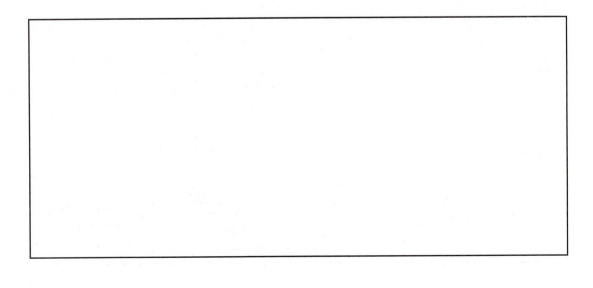

Intervention Continuum

Adjunctive	Enabling	Purposeful	Occupation-Based
Interventions that prepare for performance and participation	Interventions that focus on performance skills	Interventions that have a pre-determined goal and facilitate practice and problem solving	Interventions that are perceived as desirable, match individualized goals, and occur in appropriate context

The next step is to categorize the interventions you identified in the Intervention Brainstorm activity according to the intervention continuum. Designate the category into which each intervention falls by labeling the interventions as "A," "E," "P," or "O" to reflect them as adjunctive, enabling, purposeful, or occupation-based.

Sample Intervention Continuum

Sample interventions categorized in the intervention continuum that may be included in Becca's occupational therapy intervention plan follow.

Adjunctive Interventions	Enabling Interventions	Purposeful Interventions	Occupation-Based Interventions
Provide resources for obtaining adaptive equipment (walker bag, long-handled sponge, long-handled shoehorn, sock aid, elastic shoe laces, reacher, toilet frame, elevated toilet seat, tub bench, leg lifter). Provide handouts related to equipment use, hip precautions and restrictions, and energy conservation. Provide relaxation tape and instruction manual.	Therapist demonstrates use of adaptive equipment, precautions and restrictions, and energy conservation.	Practice dressing, bathing, bed mobility, and transfers with the use of adaptive equipment and clothes belonging to therapy clinic. Prepare and transport (using a wheeled cart) a cup of tea in the clinic kitchen and complete clean-up tasks. Stand at an elevated table to fold department clothes and towels. Stand at table to stamp and stain a leather wristband for her grandson.	Transfer, bathe, and dress using adaptive equipment in her room during her morning routine. Make hospital bed. Discuss home and community activities to facilitate problem solving of potential barriers (i.e., bus transportation, gardening, home maintenance, church activities, family events). Hang greeting cards in her room.

Session Plan—Intervention Continuum

Identify one of Becca's priority occupations:

Using interventions from the "Intervention Brainstorm," develop an occupational therapy session for Becca.

A Adjunctive Interventions	**E** Enabling Interventions	**P** Purposeful Interventions	**O** Occupation-Based Interventions

Now develop a second occupational therapy session for Becca. Consider progressing to the next session or to a session that is closer to the discontinuation of occupational therapy intervention.

Identify which of Becca's priority occupation(s) will be addressed in this session:

A Adjunctive Interventions	**E** Enabling Interventions	**P** Purposeful Interventions	**O** Occupation-Based Interventions

Sample Session Plans

Two sample session plans that may be included in Becca's occupational therapy intervention follow.

Session Plan #1

A Adjunctive Interventions	E Enabling Interventions	P Purposeful Interventions	O Occupation-Based Interventions
Provide resources for obtaining adaptive equipment (walker bag, long-handled sponge, long-handled shoehorn, sock aid, elastic shoe laces, reacher, toilet frame, elevated toilet seat, tub bench, leg lifter). *Provide handouts related to equipment use, hip precautions and restrictions, and energy conservation.*	*Therapist demonstrates use of adaptive equipment, precautions and restrictions, and energy conservation.*	*Becca practices dressing, bathing, bed mobility, and transfers with the use of adaptive equipment and clothes belonging to the therapy clinic.*	

Session Plan #2

A Adjunctive Interventions	E Enabling Interventions	P Purposeful Interventions	O Occupation-Based Interventions
		Becca prepares and transports (using a wheeled cart) a cup of tea in the clinic kitchen and completes clean-up tasks.	*Becca discusses home and community activities to facilitate problem solving of potential barriers (i.e., bus transportation, gardening, home maintenance, church activities, family events) with occupational therapy practitioner.*

Check Your Thinking 7-2

Review the sample sessions and Becca's client-centered interview. Which of Becca's priority occupations do you think the sample sessions address?

Session #1:

```



```

Session #2:

```



```

What If?

Consider how each of the following "what if?" situations would affect your intervention plan for Becca.

1. What if Becca's baseline level of functioning is different in that she ambulates with a walker, displays generalized weakness, frequently becomes short of breath, does not manage her diabetes, and has decreased range of motion in both shoulders?

2. What if Becca has macular degeneration?

3. What if Becca experiences a panic attack prior to a therapy session?

4. What if Becca's son and daughter-in-law were unable to have Becca stay with them after discharge?

CLINICAL SCENARIO #3—CHARLES

Setting:	Skilled nursing facility
Diagnosis:	Parkinson's disease
Estimated duration of intervention:	Six weeks
Anticipated discharge plan:	Home with wife and community support

Occupational Profile and Analysis of Occupational Performance

Charles is a 76-year-old retired college professor who fell at home three times in a two-day period without injury. Charles' wife, Hanna, requested an evaluation of his medication and he was admitted to an acute care hospital for three days and was subsequently transferred to a skilled nursing facility. In addition to Parkinson's disease, Charles has insulin-dependent diabetes and mild dementia, which appears to be progressing. Charles and Hanna live in a two-story home with three steps to enter. Their bathroom and bedroom are on the first floor. Prior to his hospitalization, Charles used a quad cane for getting around his home and was receiving assistance from a home health aide three times per week for bathing.

Charles is pleasant and cooperative, although he needs to be redirected in order to remain attentive to tasks and conversations. He is oriented to person and year but is unable to report the day, month, or the reason for his hospitalization. He is able to accurately recount his work history and inaccurately reports that he still drives a car. Upper extremity range of motion and strength are within normal limits bilaterally with occasional episodes of "freezing." Mild intention tremors are present in both hands, but more evident in his dominant right hand. Significant trunk rigidity is noted. Charles requires moderate assistance for bed mobility and all functional transfers. He requires minimal assistance for feeding, grooming, and upper body dressing; maximal assistance for managing his boxer shorts and pants; and total assistance to put on his socks and shoes.

Identification of Strengths and Problems

Make a list of Charles' strengths and problems based on your review of his occupational profile and analysis of occupational performance.

My List of Charles' Strengths:

My List of Charles' Problems:

Identification of Areas of Occupation, Performance Skills, Performance Patterns, and Performance Contexts

Using Appendix F, make a list of the areas of occupation, performance skills, performance patterns, and/or performance contexts that you anticipate addressing in Charles' occupational therapy intervention plan.

Client-Centered Interview Results

The following is Charles' client-centered interview, which includes a list of the occupations that he identified as needing, wanting, and being expected to perform. The occupations Charles identified as priority areas for improvement are circled.

Occupations I need to do:

1. Walk without falling

2. Feed myself

3. Get in and out of bed

4. Put my clothes on

5. Go to the bathroom by myself

Occupations I want to do:

1. Go to the golf club with my friends

2. Take care of my roses

3. Hit golf balls in my yard

4. Visit my friends and family

5. Read the newspaper

Occupations I am expected to do:

(1.) Take care of my roses

2. Pay the bills

3. Help my wife in the kitchen

4. Go to the golf club with my friends

Intervention Brainstorm

Make a list of interventions to include in Charles' occupational therapy intervention plan based on Charles' occupational profile and analysis of occupational performance, the strengths and problems you identified, and Charles' client-centered interview results.

Intervention Continuum

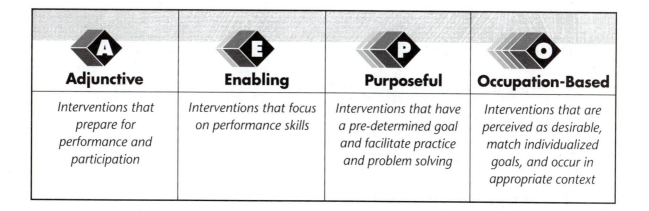

Adjunctive	**Enabling**	**Purposeful**	**Occupation-Based**
Interventions that prepare for performance and participation	*Interventions that focus on performance skills*	*Interventions that have a pre-determined goal and facilitate practice and problem solving*	*Interventions that are perceived as desirable, match individualized goals, and occur in appropriate context*

The next step is to categorize the interventions you identified in the Intervention Brainstorm activity according to the intervention continuum. Designate the category into which each intervention falls by labeling the interventions as "A," "E," "P," or "O" to reflect them as adjunctive, enabling, purposeful, or occupation-based.

Sample Intervention Continuum

Sample interventions categorized in the intervention continuum that may be included in Charles' occupational therapy intervention plan follow.

A Adjunctive Interventions	E Enabling Interventions	P Purposeful Interventions	O Occupation-Based Interventions
Provide Charles' wife with written information on caregiver body mechanics.	Upper extremity exercises using proprioceptive neuromuscular facilitation patterns. Fine motor exercises. Paper-pencil cognitive orientation activities. Instruct Charles and Hanna in safety considerations during functional mobility.	Practice transfers (i.e., bed, toilet, sofa, chair) in the clinic. Read short articles from newspaper and discuss content. Putt golf balls in the clinic.	Complete a car transfer with Charles and his wife using their vehicle. Functional ambulation to access closet, toilet, and sink during morning self-care. Transfer safely to/from bed and armchair in his room. Transport golf club, balls, and tees outside and putt golf balls in the facility courtyard.

Session Plan—Intervention Continuum

Identify one of Charles' priority occupations:

Using interventions from the "Intervention Brainstorm," develop an occupational therapy session for Charles.

Adjunctive Interventions	Enabling Interventions	Purposeful Interventions	Occupation-Based Interventions

Now develop a second occupational therapy session for Charles. Consider progressing to the next session or to a session that is closer to the discontinuation of occupational therapy intervention.

Identify which of Charles' priority occupation(s) will be addressed in this session:

Adjunctive Interventions	Enabling Interventions	Purposeful Interventions	Occupation-Based Interventions

Sample Session Plans

Two sample session plans that may be included in Charles' occupational therapy intervention follow.

Session Plan #1

A Adjunctive Interventions	**E** Enabling Interventions	**P** Purposeful Interventions	**O** Occupation-Based Interventions
Provide caregiver with written information on caregiver body mechanics.		Charles practices transfers (i.e., bed, toilet, sofa, chair) in the clinic.	Charles and Hanna perform safe transfers to/from bed and armchair in his room.

Session Plan #2

A Adjunctive Interventions	**E** Enabling Interventions	**P** Purposeful Interventions	**O** Occupation-Based Interventions
	Upper extremity exercises using proprioceptive neuromuscular facilitation patterns.	Charles putts golf balls in the clinic.	Charles transports golf club, balls, and tees outside and putts golf balls in the facility courtyard.

Check Your Thinking 7-3

Review the sample sessions and Charles' client-centered interview. Which of Charles' priority occupations do you think the sample sessions address?

Session #1:

Session #2:

What If?

Consider how each of the following "what if?" situations would affect your intervention plan for Charles.

1. What if Charles' health insurance denies continuation of therapy services before his goals are met?

2. What if Charles is frequently unsafe, remains at risk for injury, and does not understand safety precautions?

3. What if Charles requires assistance from two people for all mobility tasks and Hanna reports that she will be the only person at home with Charles?

4. What if Charles is using a wheelchair for mobility when he is discharged and the bathroom and bedroom are on the second floor of his home?

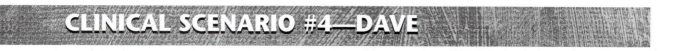

CLINICAL SCENARIO #4—DAVE

Setting:	Acute care hospital
Diagnosis:	Dementia of the Alzheimer's type
Estimated duration of intervention:	Two weeks
Anticipated discharge plan:	Return to home if possible

Occupational Profile and Analysis of Occupational Performance

Dave is a 68-year-old retired steelworker who resides with his wife, Peggy, in their two-story home. They have one married son who lives approximately 10 miles from them and is described as supportive. Peggy reports a decline in Dave's level of functioning over the last few months.

Dave is experiencing language disturbances, primarily with word finding. Dave now requires more assistance when performing his self-care tasks. Previously he was able to perform toileting, bathing, grooming, and dressing tasks with set-up and supervision, but currently requires a minimal to moderate degree of assistance. Dave continues to ambulate independently. He is displaying increased behavioral disturbances, such as wandering both during the day and night and agitation. Previously Dave assisted Peggy with light housekeeping tasks with minimal direction and assisted his son with some of the yard and garden chores. Peggy feels that she is now unable to leave Dave alone for even short periods of time. She is experiencing increased frustration due to Dave's "following (her) around the house continuously" and his sudden, unprompted outbursts of anger. Peggy reports feeling "exhausted" and is fearful that she may not be able to manage Dave in their home environment. Dave has intact motor function; however, his ability to carry out motor activities is impaired. He displays memory impairment for both new information and recall of previously learned information and disturbance in executive functioning (i.e., planning, organizing, sequencing, and abstracting).

Identification of Strengths and Problems

Make a list of Dave's strengths and problems based on your review of his occupational profile and analysis of occupational performance.

My List of Dave's Strengths:

My List of Dave's Problems:

Identification of Areas of Occupation, Performance Skills, Performance Patterns, and Performance Contexts

Using Appendix F, make a list of the areas of occupation, performance skills, performance patterns, and/or performance contexts that you anticipate addressing in Dave's occupational therapy intervention plan.

Client-Centered Interview Results

The following is Dave's client-centered interview, which includes a list of the occupations that he and his wife, Peggy, identified as needing, wanting, and expecting Dave to perform. The occupations Dave and Peggy identified as priority areas for improvement are circled.

Occupations I need to do:

1. Be as independent as possible with bathing, dressing, and feeding

(2.) Stay in one place for at least short periods of time

3. Be cooperative and follow directions

4. Go out in the community with Peggy

Occupations I want to do:

(1.) Help take care of our vegetable garden

(2.) Play with my grandchildren

3. Help Peggy around the house

4. Go bowling

5. Take walks

Occupations I am expected to do:

1. Visit with family and friends at their homes and ours

2. Interact without becoming angry for no reason

3. Not follow Peggy around all the time

4. Not leave the house without Peggy

5. Do what Peggy tells me to do

Intervention Brainstorm

Make a list of interventions to include in Dave's occupational therapy intervention plan based on Dave's occupational profile and analysis of occupational performance, the strengths and problems you identified, and Dave's client-centered interview results.

Intervention Continuum

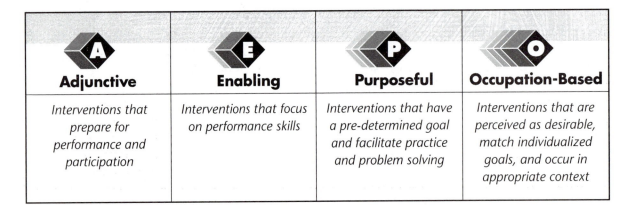

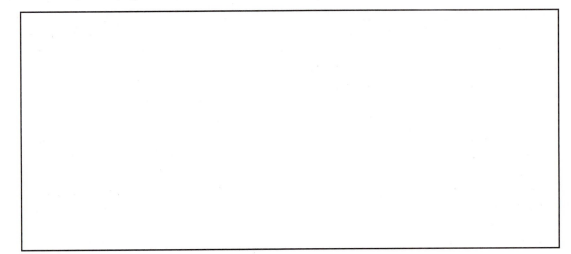			
A	**E**	**P**	**O**
Adjunctive	**Enabling**	**Purposeful**	**Occupation-Based**
Interventions that prepare for performance and participation	*Interventions that focus on performance skills*	*Interventions that have a pre-determined goal and facilitate practice and problem solving*	*Interventions that are perceived as desirable, match individualized goals, and occur in appropriate context*

The next step is to categorize the interventions you identified in the Intervention Brainstorm activity according to the intervention continuum. Designate the category into which each intervention falls by labeling the interventions as "A," "E," "P," or "O" to reflect them as adjunctive, enabling, purposeful, or occupation-based.

Sample Intervention Continuum

Sample interventions categorized in the intervention continuum that may be included in Dave's occupational therapy intervention plan follow.

Adjunctive Interventions	Enabling Interventions	Purposeful Interventions	Occupation-Based Interventions
Provide written and verbal caregiver education (i.e., understanding disease, establishing and maintaining routines, task breakdown, visual and verbal cues, behavior management strategies, caring for the caregiver, and community resources). *Provide information on assistive devices and equipment.*	*Discuss communication strategies with caregiver and client to assist with performance of daily tasks and behavior management.*	*Caregiver observes client perform self-care activities with strategies demonstrated by therapist and use of equipment (i.e., bath seat, grab bars).* *Bowling game in the clinic using plastic bowling ball and pins.* *Tabletop gardening in the clinic.* *Simple craft activities with repetitive steps.* *Play games (e.g., checkers, cards, dominoes) that require executive functioning.*	*Client and caregiver perform morning routine self-care activities in client's room using relevant strategies.* *Therapist accompanies client and caregiver to the cafeteria for lunch and facilitates use of relevant strategies.* *Collaborate with caregiver to develop a list of simple home management and leisure activities that client can perform and identify strategies for implementation.* *Develop a plan for obtaining assistive devices (e.g., monitoring devices, grab bars, tub seat, door alarms).*

Session Plan—Intervention Continuum

Identify one of Dave's priority occupations:

Using interventions from the "Intervention Brainstorm," develop an occupational therapy session for Dave.

A Adjunctive Interventions	E Enabling Interventions	P Purposeful Interventions	O Occupation-Based Interventions

Now develop a second occupational therapy session for Dave. Consider progressing to the next session or to a session that is closer to the discontinuation of occupational therapy intervention.

Identify which of Dave's priority occupation(s) will be addressed in this session:

A Adjunctive Interventions	E Enabling Interventions	P Purposeful Interventions	O Occupation-Based Interventions

Sample Session Plans

Two sample session plans that may be included in Dave's occupational therapy intervention follow.

Session Plan #1

A Adjunctive Interventions	**E** Enabling Interventions	**P** Purposeful Interventions	**O** Occupation-Based Interventions
Provide written and verbal caregiver education (i.e., understanding disease, establishing and maintaining routines, task breakdown, visual and verbal cues, behavior management strategies, caring for the caregiver, and community resources).	*Discuss communication strategies with caregiver and client to assist with performance of daily tasks and behavior management.*	*Peggy observes Dave perform self-care activities with strategies demonstrated by therapist and use of equipment (i.e., bath seat, grab bars).*	

Session Plan #2

A Adjunctive Interventions	**E** Enabling Interventions	**P** Purposeful Interventions	**O** Occupation-Based Interventions
	Discuss communication strategies with son and client to assist with performance of daily tasks and behavior management.	*Dave engages in a bowling game in the clinic using plastic bowling ball and pins with grandson.*	

Check Your Thinking 7-4

Review the sample sessions and Dave's client-centered interview. Which of Dave's priority occupations do you think the sample sessions address?

Session #1:

```

```

Session #2:

```

```

What If?

Consider how each of the following "what if?" situations would affect your intervention plan for Dave.

1. What if Dave's anticipated discharge plan is to reside at a specialized facility?

2. What if Dave falls and fractures his wrist?

3. What if Peggy sustains a back injury and her mobility and strength are restricted?

4. What if Dave is not ambulatory?

CLINICAL SCENARIO #5—GEORGE

Setting:	Home hospice
Diagnosis:	End stage cardiac disease
Estimated duration of intervention:	Six months or less
Anticipated discharge plan:	Remain in his own home

Occupational Profile and Analysis of Occupational Performance

George is a 63-year-old husband and father with end stage cardiac disease and a recent myocardial infarction. His past medical history is significant for numerous heart attacks and a stroke one year ago, which resulted in right hemiplegia. George lives with his wife, Mary, in a ranch style house with a ramp. Their only son lives across the country and they are expecting their first grandchild in six months. There is a woodworking shop in the basement that George used on a daily basis prior to his stroke. Before his most recent myocardial infarction, George required minimal assistance with self-care activities and Mary performed all home management activities. George was previously able to be alone for three to four hours at a time while his wife worked part time outside of the home. George and Mary attended religious services weekly and went out for dinner regularly. George ambulated with a quad cane and used a wheelchair for longer distances. Despite his need for minimal assistance for car transfers, George continued to drive.

At the present time, George requires minimal assistance for feeding, maximal assistance for grooming and dressing, total assistance for bathing and toileting, uses a wheelchair for household mobility, and is unable to be alone. Range of motion of his left upper extremity is within normal limits and strength is fair. Trace movement is present in his dominant right upper extremity and function of that arm is restricted to providing stabilizing assistance. George exhibits poor endurance and tires within five minutes of any type of sustained activity. No deficits in vision or hearing are apparent but decreased safety awareness is evident. George has a thorough understanding of his terminal diagnosis and "wants to make the best of a bad situation." He states that he wants "to be able to do what he did before" and also indicates that he would like to be able to go to his woodshop and "do some work."

Identification of Strengths and Problems

Make a list of George's strengths and problems based on your review of his occupational profile and analysis of occupational performance.

My List of George's Strengths:

My List of George's Problems:

Identification of Areas of Occupation, Performance Skills, Performance Patterns, and Performance Contexts

Using Appendix F, make a list of the areas of occupation, performance skills, performance patterns, and/or performance contexts that you anticipate addressing in George's occupational therapy intervention plan.

Client-Centered Interview Results

The following is George's client-centered interview, which includes a list of the occupations that he and his wife, Mary, identified as needing, wanting, and expecting George to perform. The occupations George and Mary identified as priority areas for improvement are circled.

Occupations I need to do:

1. Get dressed and bathed by myself

2. Use the bathroom without help

3. Walk around the house by myself

4. Stay alone at home while my wife is at work

Occupations I want to do:

(1.) Make a rocking horse for my future grandchild

2. Go to church and out for dinner with my wife

3. Talk to my son on the phone

Occupations I am expected to do:

1. Stay alone in the house while my wife is at work

2. Stay involved with church activities

3. Help my wife with housework

Intervention Brainstorm

Make a list of interventions to include in George's occupational therapy intervention plan based on George's occupational profile and analysis of occupational performance, the strengths and problems you identified, and George's client-centered interview results.

Intervention Continuum

A Adjunctive	**E** Enabling	**P** Purposeful	**O** Occupation-Based
Interventions that prepare for performance and participation	*Interventions that focus on performance skills*	*Interventions that have a pre-determined goal and facilitate practice and problem solving*	*Interventions that are perceived as desirable, match individualized goals, and occur in appropriate context*

The next step is to categorize the interventions you identified in the Intervention Brainstorm activity according to the intervention continuum. Designate the category into which each intervention falls by labeling the interventions as "A," "E," "P," or "O" to reflect them as adjunctive, enabling, purposeful, or occupation-based.

Sample Intervention Continuum

Sample interventions categorized in the intervention continuum that may be included in George's occupational therapy intervention plan follow.

Adjunctive Interventions	Enabling Interventions	Purposeful Interventions	Occupation-Based Interventions
Provide written information on energy conservation and safety issues. Recruit a hospice volunteer to help during woodworking activities.	Provide education and demonstration of energy conservation. Discuss and problem solve safety practices related to woodworking activities. Exercise to build endurance and standing tolerance.	Practice transfers from a variety of surfaces inside and outside the home. Use energy conservation strategies while engaged in self-care training during his therapy session. Retrieve and transport items between the refrigerator and microwave.	Incorporate energy conservation techniques while performing activities of daily living retraining at "real" times. Incorporate safety precautions while engaged in woodworking task. Use energy conservation strategies as he shows therapist to the door following the therapy session. Therapist supervises George and the volunteer during woodworking session, and provides cues to incorporate and reinforce safety, energy conservation, one-handed techniques, and ergonomic strategies.

Session Plan—Intervention Continuum

Identify one of George's priority occupations:

Using interventions from the "Intervention Brainstorm," develop an occupational therapy session for George.

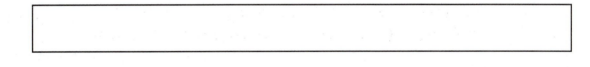

Adjunctive Interventions	Enabling Interventions	Purposeful Interventions	Occupation-Based Interventions

Now develop a second occupational therapy session for George. Consider progressing to the next session or to a session that is closer to the discontinuation of occupational therapy intervention.

Identify which of George's priority occupation(s) will be addressed in this session:

Adjunctive Interventions	Enabling Interventions	Purposeful Interventions	Occupation-Based Interventions

Sample Session Plans

Two sample session plans that may be included in George's occupational therapy intervention follow.

Session Plan #1

A **Adjunctive Interventions**	E **Enabling Interventions**	P **Purposeful Interventions**	O **Occupation-Based Interventions**
Provide written information on energy conservation and safety issues.	*Provide education and demonstration of energy conservation.*	*George uses energy conservation strategies while engaged in self-care training during his therapy session.*	*George uses energy conservation strategies as he shows therapist to the door following the therapy session.*

Session Plan #2

A **Adjunctive Interventions**	E **Enabling Interventions**	P **Purposeful Interventions**	O **Occupation-Based Interventions**
Recruit hospice volunteer to help during woodworking activities.			*Therapist supervises George, and the volunteer during woodworking session, and provides cues to incorporate and reinforce safety, energy conservation, one-handed techniques, and ergonomic strategies.*

Check Your Thinking 7-5

Review the sample sessions and George's client-centered interview. Which of George's priority occupations do you think the sample sessions address?

Session #1:

```

```

Session #2:

```

```

What If?

Consider how each of the following "what if?" situations would affect your intervention plan for George.

1. What if George is unable to gain enough strength and endurance to be able to negotiate the stairs to his woodshop?

2. What if George has no desire to regain his previous occupational role of being a woodworker? How would you help George identify alternate occupational roles?

3. What if you are unable to find a volunteer who is willing to work with George?

4. What if George became tearful during a therapy session and indicated that he felt useless and wished he would "just die?"

CLINICAL SCENARIO #6—JEAN

Setting:	Long-term care facility
Diagnoses:	Chronic obstructive pulmonary disease; nonoperable hernia; generalized weakness; degenerative joint disease; morbid obesity; recent pneumonia; and bowel obstruction
Estimated duration of intervention:	Three times per week for two weeks
Anticipated discharge plan:	Continue residence in long-term care facility and refer to restorative nursing program

Occupational Profile and Analysis of Occupational Performance

Jean is an 82-year-old, single woman who resides in a long-term care facility and was recently hospitalized for three weeks due to pneumonia and a bowel obstruction. The facility staff reports that Jean loves to read, take care of people, follow the local sports teams on television and radio, garden, and socialize with family and friends. Jean is nonambulatory and propels her wheelchair using both lower extremities. Prior to her most recent hospitalization, the Minimum Data Set revealed that Jean was independent in basic activities of daily living. She typically bathed herself using an extended tub bench and handheld shower, used a raised commode and wall-mounted grab bar for toileting, and propelled herself to the dining room for meals. She wore housedresses and slip-on shoes for ease in dressing. Jean typically left her room at 9:00 A.M. and attended multiple social and religious activities in the building.

Upon return to the facility Jean's hearing, vision, cognition, and bilateral upper extremity function are within normal limits. Her endurance is decreased. She is able to propel herself in her wheelchair only one-third of the way around the interior of the building prior to experiencing shortness of breath. Jean had been able to complete a minimum of one lap with ease prior to her hospitalization. Jean currently chooses to stay in her room for lunch, as she cannot transport herself to the dining room. She requires minimal assistance for all functional transfers. She is unable to reach her lower legs and feet without becoming short of breath and, therefore, requires assistance with lower body dressing and bathing. Jean has had occupational therapy intervention in the past and is knowledgeable of energy conservation and work simplification strategies.

Identification of Strengths and Problems

Make a list of Jean's strengths and problems based on your review of her occupational profile and analysis of occupational performance.

My List of Jean's Strengths:

┌───┐
│ **My List of Jean's Problems:**   │
│   │
│   │
│   │
│   │
│   │
└───┘

Identification of Areas of Occupation, Performance Skills, Performance Patterns, and Performance Contexts

Using Appendix F, make a list of the areas of occupation, performance skills, performance patterns, and/or performance contexts that you anticipate addressing in Jean's occupational therapy intervention plan.

┌───┐
│   │
│   │
│   │
│   │
│   │
│   │
│   │
└───┘

Client-Centered Interview Results

The following is Jean's client-centered interview, which includes a list of the occupations that she identified as needing, wanting, and being expected to perform. The occupations Jean identified as priority areas for improvement are circled.

Occupations I need to do:

1. Call my daughter every day

②. Do more for myself

③. Eat my meals in the dining room with my friends

4. Plan how I do things better

Occupations I want to do:

(1.) Take care of myself

(2.) Go to more social activities

3. Be with other people and not be alone

(4.) Be in close contact with my family and friends

5. Do more for myself

Occupations I am expected to do:

1. Pay my bills

2. Be reasonable and treat other people who live here, as well as staff, with respect

3. Keep the noise down in my room so as not to disturb my roommate

4. Do more for myself

Intervention Brainstorm

Make a list of interventions to include in Jean's occupational therapy intervention plan based on Jean's occupational profile and analysis of occupational performance, the strengths and problems you identified, and Jean's client-centered interview results.

Intervention Continuum

◀A▶ Adjunctive	◀E▶ Enabling	◀P▶ Purposeful	◀O▶ Occupation-Based
Interventions that prepare for performance and participation	*Interventions that focus on performance skills*	*Interventions that have a pre-determined goal and facilitate practice and problem solving*	*Interventions that are perceived as desirable, match individualized goals, and occur in appropriate context*

The next step is to categorize the interventions you identified in the Intervention Brainstorm activity according to the intervention continuum. Designate the category into which each intervention falls by labeling the interventions as "A," "E," "P," or "O" to reflect them as adjunctive, enabling, purposeful, or occupation-based.

Sample Intervention Continuum

Sample interventions categorized in the intervention continuum that may be included in Jean's occupational therapy intervention plan follow.

Adjunctive Interventions	Enabling Interventions	Purposeful Interventions	Occupation-Based Interventions
Introduce long-handled dressing equipment for possible use with lower extremity dressing and bathing.	Provide a daily schedule for the next week outlining each day's activities and level of activity participation that will increase her endurance and socialization. Review energy conservation and work simplification literature and modify daily schedule as needed. Demonstrate long-handled dressing equipment for possible use with lower extremity dressing and bathing. Self-propel wheelchair one-half lap of inside perimeter of building using bilateral lower extremities, taking rest breaks and incorporating energy conservation/work simplification.	Practice transfers to and from wheelchair, bed, commode, tub bench, armchair, and recliner chair in the therapy clinic. Use pursed-lip breathing techniques while negotiating obstacles in the clinic. Practice using long-handled dressing equipment for lower extremity dressing and bathing during afternoon therapy session.	Transfer to extended tub bench in her room and complete her own bathing. Complete toileting, including transfer, in the facility's public restroom near activities room and dining room that she would typically use during the day. Propel self to dining room while incorporating energy conservation and work simplification principles after initiating plans with friends to eat lunch and dinner meals in dining room. Deliver mail to residents' rooms using wheelchair while incorporating energy conservation and work simplification principles with assistance and cues from therapist as needed.

Session Plan—Intervention Continuum

Identify one of Jean's priority occupations:

Using interventions from the "Intervention Brainstorm," develop an occupational therapy session for Jean.

Adjunctive Interventions	Enabling Interventions	Purposeful Interventions	Occupation-Based Interventions

Now develop a second occupational therapy session for Jean. Consider progressing to the next session or to a session that is closer to the discontinuation of occupational therapy intervention.

Identify which of Jean's priority occupation(s) will be addressed in this session:

Adjunctive Interventions	Enabling Interventions	Purposeful Interventions	Occupation-Based Interventions

Sample Session Plans

Two sample session plans that may be included in Jean's occupational therapy intervention follow.

Session Plan #1

Adjunctive Interventions	Enabling Interventions	Purposeful Interventions	Occupation-Based Interventions
Introduce long-handled dressing equipment for possible use with lower extremity dressing and bathing.	Demonstrate long-handled dressing equipment for possible use with lower extremity dressing and bathing.	Jean practices using long-handled dressing equipment for lower extremity dressing and bathing during afternoon therapy session.	

Session Plan #2

Adjunctive Interventions	Enabling Interventions	Purposeful Interventions	Occupation-Based Interventions
	Self-propel wheelchair one-half lap of inside perimeter of building using bilateral lower extremities, taking rest breaks and incorporating energy conservation/work simplification.		Jean propels self to dining room while incorporating energy conservation and work simplification principles after initiating plans with friends to eat lunch and dinner meals in dining room.

Check Your Thinking 7-6

Review the sample sessions and Jean's client-centered interview. Which of Jean's priority occupations do you think the sample sessions address?

Session #1:

```



```

Session #2:

```
┌─────────────────────────────────────────────────────────────────────┐
│                                                                       │
│                                                                       │
│                                                                       │
└─────────────────────────────────────────────────────────────────────┘
```

What If?

Consider how each of the following "what if?" situations would affect your intervention plan for Jean.

1. What if Jean is able to ambulate?

2. What if Jean lives at home with her daughter?

3. What if Jean is diagnosed with dementia?

4. What if Jean is a loner and prefers not to be around other people?

CLINICAL SCENARIO #7—KAY

Setting:	Assisted living facility
Diagnoses:	Cerebrovascular accident; major depression
Estimated duration of intervention:	Two months
Anticipated discharge plan:	Home to live alone

Occupational Profile and Analysis of Occupational Performance

Kay is a 66-year-old, widowed female who recently suffered a right-sided temporal bleed with left-sided weakness. She was hospitalized in an acute care hospital for four days; was transferred to the rehabilitation unit for two weeks; and then was discharged to an assisted living facility. Because she requires assistance to ambulate she is unable to return home alone. However, she hopes to eventually return to her home, a one-story house with laundry facilities in the basement.

Upon evaluation, Kay is noted to have left-sided neglect with moderate homonymous hemianopsia. She is alert and oriented but displays impulsivity during performance of her daily occupations. She has full active range of motion in her left shoulder and elbow with fair strength, and limited movement in her wrist and hand. Her right upper extremity function is good. Kay requires minimal assistance for grooming and upper body dressing and moderate assistance for lower body dressing. She transfers with minimal assistance because of impulsivity. Kay currently displays a flat affect, poor eye contact, and frequently isolates herself from staff and the other residents. She does not initiate interactions and her responses upon direct approach are limited to a few words. Prior to her hospitalization, Kay completed all basic and instrumental activities of daily living independently, including driving. She reportedly visited her daughter and granddaughter on a weekly basis.

Identification of Strengths and Problems

Make a list of Kay's strengths and problems based on your review of her occupational profile and analysis of occupational performance.

My List of Kay's Strengths:

My List of Kay's Problems:

Identification of Areas of Occupation, Performance Skills, Performance Patterns, and Performance Contexts

Using Appendix F, make a list of the areas of occupation, performance skills, performance patterns, and/or performance contexts that you anticipate addressing in Kay's occupational therapy intervention plan.

Client-Centered Interview Results

The following is Kay's client-centered interview, which includes a list of the occupations that she identified as needing, wanting, and being expected to perform. The occupations Kay identified as priority areas for improvement are circled.

Occupations I need to do:

(1.) Dress myself

(2.) Walk around my house

3. Get my arm working again

4. Make telephone calls

5. Drive my car to the store and my daughter's home

Occupations I want to do:

1. Go to bingo

(2.) Visit my daughter and granddaughter

(3.) Cook one meal each day

(4.) Go home

Occupations I am expected to do:

1. Pay my bills

2. Clean my house

3. Do my laundry

4. Baby-sit for my granddaughter

Intervention Brainstorm

Make a list of interventions to include in Kay's occupational therapy intervention plan based on Kay's occupational profile and analysis of occupational performance, the strengths and problems you identified, and Kay's client-centered interview results.

Intervention Continuum

Adjunctive	**Enabling**	**Purposeful**	**Occupation-Based**
Interventions that prepare for performance and participation	Interventions that focus on performance skills	Interventions that have a pre-determined goal and facilitate practice and problem solving	Interventions that are perceived as desirable, match individualized goals, and occur in appropriate context

The next step is to categorize the interventions you identified in the Intervention Brainstorm activity according to the intervention continuum. Designate the category into which each intervention falls by labeling the interventions as "A," "E," "P," or "O" to reflect them as adjunctive, enabling, purposeful, or occupation-based.

Sample Intervention Continuum

Sample interventions categorized in the intervention continuum that may be included in Kay's occupational therapy intervention plan follow.

A **Adjunctive Interventions**	**E** **Enabling Interventions**	**P** **Purposeful Interventions**	**O** **Occupation-Based Interventions**
Provide elastic shoelaces and a walker bag. *Provide a catalog of one-handed equipment resources.*	*Self range of motion exercises for the left wrist and hand.* *Weight-bearing activities with left hand and wrist.* *Paper-pencil scanning exercises (i.e., circling the "x").* *Practice one-handed buttoning and zippering on a dressing board.*	*Complete word searches, crossword puzzles, and bingo game using compensation strategies for left neglect.* *Ambulate with hemi-walker through doors, opening and closing, using a key, etc.* *Verbalize and practice steps in hemi-dressing techniques using a clinic shirt during a therapy session.* *Practice cutting a piece of fruit or vegetable with a cutting board and a rocker knife and discuss related safety precautions.*	*Participate in a home visit with therapist and daughter.* *Invite daughter to have lunch with her in the kitchenette and prepare a simple meal while incorporating one-handed techniques and neglect strategies.*

Session Plan—Intervention Continuum

Identify one of Kay's priority occupations:

Using interventions from the "Intervention Brainstorm," develop an occupational therapy session for Kay.

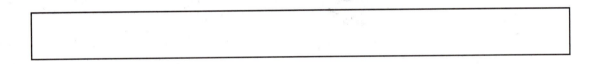 Adjunctive Interventions	Enabling Interventions	Purposeful Interventions	Occupation-Based Interventions

Now develop a second occupational therapy session for Kay. Consider progressing to the next session or to a session that is closer to the discontinuation of occupational therapy intervention.

Identify which of Kay's priority occupation(s) will be addressed in this session:

Adjunctive Interventions	Enabling Interventions	Purposeful Interventions	Occupation-Based Interventions

Sample Session Plans

Two sample session plans that may be included in Kay's occupational therapy intervention follow.

Session Plan #1

A Adjunctive Interventions	E Enabling Interventions	P Purposeful Interventions	O Occupation-Based Interventions
Provide a catalog of one-handed equipment resources.	Kay practices one-handed buttoning and zippering on a dressing board.	Kay verbalizes and practices steps in hemi-dressing techniques using a clinic shirt during a therapy session.	

Session Plan #2

A Adjunctive Interventions	E Enabling Interventions	P Purposeful Interventions	O Occupation-Based Interventions
			Kay invites her daughter to have lunch with her in the kitchenette and prepares a simple meal while incorporating one-handed techniques and neglect strategies.

Check Your Thinking 7-7

Review the sample sessions and Kay's client-centered interview. Which of Kay's priority occupations do you think the sample sessions address?

Session #1:

Session #2:

What If?

Consider how each of the following "what if?" situations would affect your intervention plan for Kay.

1. What if Kay's daughter reports suspecting Kay of abusing alcohol?

2. What if Kay's status remains unchanged and she is unable to return home independently?

3. What if Kay develops a deep vein thrombosis and is temporarily confined to bed?

4. What if Kay develops reflex sympathetic dystrophy/complex regional pain syndrome in her left arm?

CLINICAL SCENARIO #8—MAURA

Setting:	Second-grade classroom
Diagnoses:	Learning disability and attention deficit/hyperactivity disorder
Estimated duration of intervention:	School year
Anticipated discharge plan:	Regular education classroom with learning support

Occupational Profile and Analysis of Occupational Performance

Maura is an 8-year-old whose conditions have recently been diagnosed. She is fully included in her second-grade classroom, but receives math instruction in the Learning Support Classroom. Maura's teacher describes her as having strengths in reading and science. Areas of concern for Maura include sloppy handwriting, difficulty sitting still in the classroom (i.e., constant fidgeting and chewing on pencils), and inability to get along with peers. Maura states that her favorite subjects in school are reading and gym, with her least favorite subjects being art and writing. Maura's mother describes her as an active child. At home, her chores include making her bed, setting and clearing the table, and feeding the cat. Maura is able to ride a bicycle, ice skate, and roller blade. Maura's mother reports she has difficulty maintaining friendships.

Maura's gross motor skills are age appropriate. She demonstrates adequate muscle tone, strength, and endurance for functional tasks. Maura is able to hop, skip, dribble a ball, perform jumping jacks, and jump rope. During recess, Maura plays alone, either swinging or climbing on the playground equipment. Maura manages small buttons and ties her shoes independently. Maura grasps her pencil tightly in her fist, using a "hook" type grasp with a flexed wrist, and presses hard on her paper when writing. Her printed work reveals difficulty with letter formation, alignment on the writing line, and spacing. She has difficulty remembering how to make the letters. Maura seeks out a variety of intense sensory input throughout the day.

Identification of Strengths and Problems

Make a list of Maura's strengths and problems based on your review of her occupational profile and analysis of occupational performance.

My List of Maura's Strengths:

My List of Maura's Problems:

Identification of Areas of Occupation, Performance Skills, Performance Patterns, and Performance Contexts

Using Appendix F, make a list of the areas of occupation, performance skills, performance patterns, and/or performance contexts that you anticipate addressing in Maura's occupational therapy intervention plan.

Client-Centered Interview Results

The following is Maura's client-centered interview, which includes a list of the occupations that she and her parents identified as needing, wanting, and expecting Maura to perform. The occupations Maura and her parents identified as priority areas for improvement are circled.

Occupations I need to do:

1. Be nice to my friends

2. Print so the teacher can read it

3. Not press so hard with my pencil

4. Stay in my seat in the classroom

5. Work slowly

Occupations I want to do:

(1.) Learn to print neater

(2.) Play with other kids

(3.) Get a good report from my teacher

(4.) Be a famous ice skater

(5.) Get stars on my school chart

Occupations I am expected to do:

1. Do my jobs at home and at school

2. Do my homework

3. Listen to my teacher

4. Get a good report card

5. Be nice to my little brother

Intervention Brainstorm

Make a list of interventions to include in Maura's occupational therapy intervention plan based on Maura's occupational profile and analysis of occupational performance, the strengths and problems you identified, and Maura's client-centered interview results.

Intervention Continuum

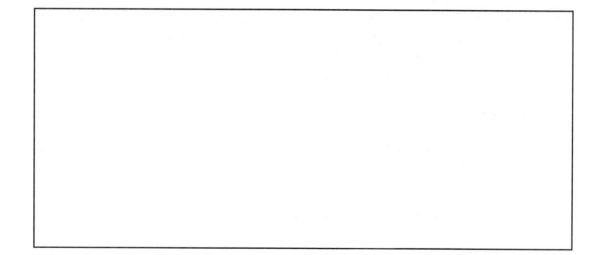

A	E	P	O
Adjunctive	**Enabling**	**Purposeful**	**Occupation-Based**
Interventions that prepare for performance and participation	*Interventions that focus on performance skills*	*Interventions that have a pre-determined goal and facilitate practice and problem solving*	*Interventions that are perceived as desirable, match individualized goals, and occur in appropriate context*

The next step is to categorize the interventions you identified in the Intervention Brainstorm activity according to the intervention continuum. Designate the category into which each intervention falls by labeling the interventions as "A," "E," "P," or "O" to reflect them as adjunctive, enabling, purposeful, or occupation-based.

Sample Intervention Continuum

Sample interventions categorized in the intervention continuum that may be included in Maura's occupational therapy intervention plan follow.

(A) Adjunctive Interventions	(E) Enabling Interventions	(P) Purposeful Interventions	(O) Occupation-Based Interventions
Provide sensory integration in-service to teachers.	Hand warm-ups in preparation for writing (seat push-ups, squeeze a ball, thumb-to-finger touching).	Use a vibrating pen to complete mazes.	Participate in wheelbarrow races, traffic cone obstacle course, and sack races during "Olympic Day" at school.
Provide a letter strip on desk for proper paper slant.	Try different strategies for self-regulation (movement, tactile, oral, etc.) and begin to identify which ones help Maura feel calm and focused.	Play tic-tac-toe (with another student) on the chalkboard using a small piece of chalk.	Write a short paragraph describing her feelings and thoughts about "Olympic Day" to be included in the class newsletter.
Discuss the need to incorporate sensory breaks into schedule with teacher.	Complete exercises to "get the wiggles out" and get Maura ready for handwriting.		Provide instruction for proper letter formation, paper positioning, and introduce finger spacing before Maura writes out her spelling words.
	Trace letters in carpet squares and replicate letters with waxed string.		Create a "special occasion" card for her brother using a mechanical pencil to reinforce pencil pressure.

Session Plan—Intervention Continuum

Identify one of Maura's priority occupations:

```
┌─────────────────────────────────────────────────────────────────────┐
│                                                                       │
│                                                                       │
│                                                                       │
└─────────────────────────────────────────────────────────────────────┘
```

Using interventions from the "Intervention Brainstorm," develop an occupational therapy session for Maura.

Adjunctive Interventions	Enabling Interventions	Purposeful Interventions	Occupation-Based Interventions

Now develop a second occupational therapy session for Maura. Consider progressing to the next session or to a session that is closer to the discontinuation of occupational therapy intervention.

Identify which of Maura's priority occupation(s) will be addressed in this session:

```
┌─────────────────────────────────────────────────────────────────────┐
│                                                                       │
│                                                                       │
│                                                                       │
└─────────────────────────────────────────────────────────────────────┘
```

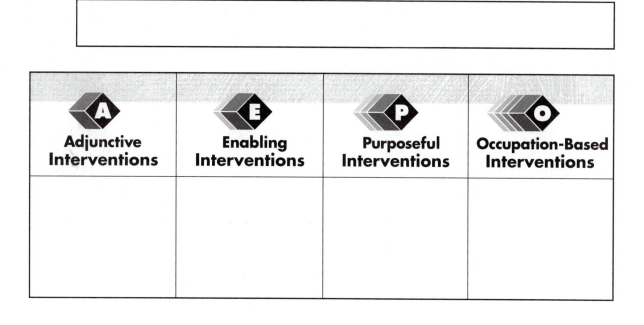

Adjunctive Interventions	Enabling Interventions	Purposeful Interventions	Occupation-Based Interventions

Sample Session Plans

Two sample session plans that may be included in Maura's occupational therapy intervention follow.

Session Plan #1

A Adjunctive Interventions	**E** Enabling Interventions	**P** Purposeful Interventions	**O** Occupation-Based Interventions
Provide a letter strip on desk for proper paper slant.	*Hand warm-ups in preparation for writing (seat push-ups, squeeze a ball, thumb-to-finger touching).* *Complete exercises to "get the wiggles out" and get Maura ready for handwriting.*		*Maura creates a "special occasion" card for her brother using a mechanical pencil to reinforce pencil pressure.*

Session Plan #2

A Adjunctive Interventions	**E** Enabling Interventions	**P** Purposeful Interventions	**O** Occupation-Based Interventions
			Therapist assists Maura as she participates in wheelbarrow races, traffic cone obstacle course, and sack races during "Olympic Day" at school.

Check Your Thinking 7-8

Review the sample sessions and Maura's client-centered interview. Which of Maura's priority occupations do you think the sample sessions address?

Session #1:

```
[                                                              ]
```

Session #2:

```
[                                                              ]
```

What If?

Consider how each of the following "what if?" situations would affect your intervention plan for Maura.

1. What if Maura's teacher feels that Maura is too much of a distraction to the other students and asked you to provide occupational therapy intervention outside of the classroom?

2. What if Maura's parents ask you to provide occupational therapy intervention in their home?

3. What if Maura's disruptive behaviors increase and she is hitting other students and calling them names?

4. What if Maura has self-abusive behaviors?

CLINICAL SCENARIO #9—MIGUEL

Setting:	Inpatient rehabilitation facility
Diagnosis:	C5 tetraplegia, complete
Estimated duration of intervention:	Three months
Anticipated discharge plan:	Home with parents

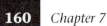

Occupational Profile and Analysis of Occupational Performance

Miguel is a 20-year-old college junior who sustained a spinal cord injury as a result of a diving accident three weeks ago. Miguel lives with his parents and younger sister in a two-story home with four steps to enter. The bedroom and bathroom are on the second floor. Miguel's mother is a teacher and his father is a self-employed carpenter who has already initiated plans for constructing a ramp and an addition to the family home. He has a large circle of friends and a girlfriend of three years who is studying abroad. Miguel is an engineering major with a minor in computer programming at a local university to which he commuted with his friends.

Miguel is quiet during his occupational therapy evaluation but provides accurate information about his home, hobbies, and daily activities. There is no evidence of visual, hearing, or cognitive deficits. Strength of the residual C5 musculature is fair, with trace C6 muscle activity; sensation is intact through C5, impaired at C6, and absent at C7 and below. Miguel is currently using a manual wheelchair and is dependent for wheelchair mobility and all self-care activities. He has bilateral palmer splints, a wrist cock-up splint for his dominant right hand, and a universal cuff that were issued at the trauma center from which he was transferred. Miguel reports that he initiated self-feeding training at the trauma center with the occupational therapist but that he still "needs a lot of help." Miguel states that he understands the implications of his injury, but further notes that he is hopeful that he will be able to use his hands and walk in the future.

Identification of Strengths and Problems

Make a list of Miguel's strengths and problems based on your review of his occupational profile and analysis of occupational performance.

My List of Miguel's Strengths:

My List of Miguel's Problems:

Identification of Areas of Occupation, Performance Skills, Performance Patterns, and Performance Contexts

Using Appendix F, make a list of the areas of occupation, performance skills, performance patterns, and/or performance contexts that you anticipate addressing in Miguel's occupational therapy intervention plan.

Client-Centered Interview Results

The following is Miguel's client-centered interview, which includes a list of the occupations that he identified as needing, wanting, and being expected to perform. The occupations Miguel identified as priority areas for improvement are circled.

Occupations I need to do:

(1.) Go back to school

2. Drive

(3.) Take care of myself

(4.) Walk

(5.) Use my computer

Occupations I want to do:

(1.) Use my hands

2. Walk

3. Have a relationship with my girlfriend

4. Finish school

Occupations I am expected to do:

1. Finish school

2. Get a job

3. Do things for myself

Intervention Brainstorm

Make a list of interventions to include in Miguel's occupational therapy intervention plan based on Miguel's occupational profile and analysis of occupational performance, the strengths and problems you identified, and Miguel's client-centered interview results.

Intervention Continuum

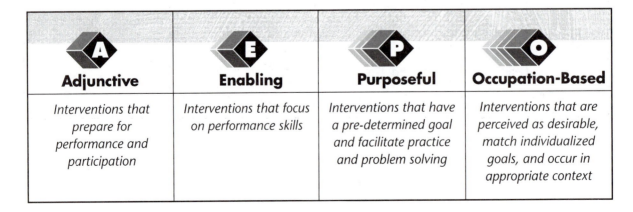

Adjunctive	Enabling	Purposeful	Occupation-Based
Interventions that prepare for performance and participation	Interventions that focus on performance skills	Interventions that have a pre-determined goal and facilitate practice and problem solving	Interventions that are perceived as desirable, match individualized goals, and occur in appropriate context

The next step is to categorize the interventions you identified in the Intervention Brainstorm activity according to the intervention continuum. Designate the category into which each intervention falls by labeling the interventions as "A," "E," "P," or "O" to reflect them as adjunctive, enabling, purposeful, or occupation-based.

Sample Intervention Continuum

Sample interventions categorized in the intervention continuum that may be included in Miguel's occupational therapy intervention plan follow.

A Adjunctive Interventions	E Enabling Interventions	P Purposeful Interventions	O Occupation-Based Interventions
Provide information related to home modifications, adaptive equipment, and electronic aids to daily living (e.g., voice recognition software for computer). *Upper extremity passive range of motion.*	*Active assistive, active, and progressive resistive upper extremity exercises.* *Practice manipulating and positioning feeding utensils using inedible objects (i.e., clay).* *Provide instruction and discuss the use of electronic aids to daily living with repeat demonstration.* *Use mouse input device to move the cursor to a variety of locations on the computer screen.*	*Practice use of computer input equipment by copying written text.* *Make a telephone call for weather or time check using switch input to access the telephone.* *Self feed with an adapted spoon during his therapy session.* *Type his name and address using the mouse, and keyboard input devices, and voice recognition software.*	*Eat dinner with family in hospital cafeteria using adaptive equipment with instruction and supervision from therapist.* *Write a letter to his girlfriend using voice recognition software, mouse, and keyboard input devices.*

Session Plan—Intervention Continuum

Identify one of Miguel's priority occupations:

Using interventions from the "Intervention Brainstorm," develop an occupational therapy session for Miguel.

A Adjunctive Interventions	**E** Enabling Interventions	**P** Purposeful Interventions	**O** Occupation-Based Interventions

Now develop a second occupational therapy session for Miguel. Consider progressing to the next session or to a session that is closer to the discontinuation of occupational therapy intervention.

Identify which of Miguel's priority occupation(s) will be addressed in this session:

A Adjunctive Interventions	**E** Enabling Interventions	**P** Purposeful Interventions	**O** Occupation-Based Interventions

Sample Session Plans

Two sample session plans that may be included in Miguel's occupational therapy intervention follow.

Session Plan #1

A Adjunctive Interventions	E Enabling Interventions	P Purposeful Interventions	O Occupation-Based Interventions
	Use mouse input device to move the cursor to a variety of locations on the computer screen.	*Miguel practices use of computer input equipment by copying written text.*	*Miguel writes a letter to his girlfriend using voice recognition software, mouse, and keyboard input devices.*

Session Plan #2

A Adjunctive Interventions	E Enabling Interventions	P Purposeful Interventions	O Occupation-Based Interventions
Upper extremity passive range of motion.	*Practice manipulating and positioning feeding utensils using inedible objects (i.e., clay).*	*Miguel feeds himself with an adapted spoon during his therapy session.*	

Check Your Thinking 7-9

Review the sample sessions and Miguel's client-centered interview. Which of Miguel's priority occupations do you think the sample sessions address?

Session #1:

Session #2:

What If?

Consider how each of the following "what if?" situations would affect your intervention plan for Miguel.

1. What if Miguel develops a decubitus ulcer and is on limited sitting status?

2. What if Miguel sustained a head injury in addition to the spinal cord injury?

3. What if Miguel's injury level is C4 and he has no voluntary movement of his upper extremities?

4. What if Miguel's family is in the process of relocating to another state due to a change in his father's employment?

CLINICAL SCENARIO #10—PAM

Setting:	Outpatient hand clinic
Diagnosis:	Carpal tunnel syndrome
Estimated duration of intervention:	Four visits, one visit per week
Anticipated discharge plan:	Continue with independent living

Occupational Profile and Analysis of Occupational Performance

Pam is a single, 42-year-old full-time clerk for a major mail order company where she receives and enters customer orders into the computer system. Pam has intermittently experienced tingling sensations at night in both hands over the past year. She has ignored these symptoms until recently when she was awakened with "shooting" pains in her right fingers, wrist, and forearm. Despite the discomfort, she went to work and played racquetball that evening. At her doctor visit two weeks later, she was diagnosed with carpal tunnel syndrome and the doctor recommended a surgical release. At Pam's request, the doctor agreed to try a conservative treatment approach and referred her to occupational therapy at an outpatient clinic.

Pam describes herself as an "active and independent" person who "works, plays racquetball, and bikes." Pam states that therapy is a "last-ditch" effort in an attempt to avoid surgery, which she anticipates would interfere with her lifestyle. She is right-hand dominant with normal upper extremity active range of motion and strength, including bilateral grip strengths that are above the 90th percentile for her age and gender. She describes the sensation in her right wrist and hand as feeling "swollen inside" although there is no observable swelling or objective differences in volumetric measures. Pam reports that she occasionally has "trouble making her fingers work" and provides examples related to using her computer keyboard effectively, managing small buttons, and manipulating her car keys. She also states that her hands frequently "ache" during her workday, and at night she experiences pain between "8 and 10" on a 10-point scale. She has positive Tinel and Phalen signs in the right thumb and index finger.

Identification of Strengths and Problems

Make a list of Pam's strengths and problems based on your review of her occupational profile and analysis of occupational performance.

My List of Pam's Strengths:

My List of Pam's Problems:

Identification of Areas of Occupation, Performance Skills, Performance Patterns, and Performance Contexts

Using Appendix F, make a list of the areas of occupation, performance skills, performance patterns, and/or performance contexts that you anticipate addressing in Pam's occupational therapy intervention plan.

Client-Centered Interview Results

The following is Pam's client-centered interview, which includes a list of the occupations that she identified as needing, wanting, and being expected to perform. The occupations Pam identified as priority areas for improvement are circled.

Occupations I need to do:

(1.) Continue to work

(2.) Make time for these therapy visits and exercises to avoid surgery

3. Grocery shop and run other errands

4. Cook

5. Clean my apartment

Occupations I want to do:

(1.) Play racquetball and bike

(2.) Be able to do my normal routine, without pain

3. Stay connected with my friends

Occupations I am expected to do:

1. Show up for tournament games

2. Be productive at work

3. Train new employees

Intervention Brainstorm

Make a list of interventions to include in Pam's occupational therapy intervention plan based on Pam's occupational profile and analysis of occupational performance, the strengths and problems you identified, and Pam's client-centered interview results.

Intervention Continuum

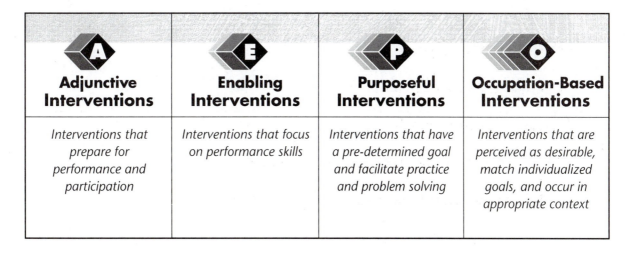

Adjunctive Interventions	Enabling Interventions	Purposeful Interventions	Occupation-Based Interventions
Interventions that prepare for performance and participation	*Interventions that focus on performance skills*	*Interventions that have a pre-determined goal and facilitate practice and problem solving*	*Interventions that are perceived as desirable, match individualized goals, and occur in appropriate context*

The next step is to categorize the interventions you identified in the Intervention Brainstorm activity according to the intervention continuum. Designate the category into which each intervention falls by labeling the interventions as "A," "E," "P," or "O" to reflect them as adjunctive, enabling, purposeful, or occupation-based.

Sample Intervention Continuum

Sample interventions categorized in the intervention continuum that may be included in Pam's occupational therapy intervention plan follow.

A Adjunctive Interventions	E Enabling Interventions	P Purposeful Interventions	O Occupation-Based Interventions
Issue brochure describing pathology and prevention strategies.	*Fine motor exercises.*	*Practice lifting items of various sizes, shapes, and weights while incorporating prevention strategies.*	*Bring racquetball racquet to therapy for grip and form assessment and therapist recommendations for modifications.*
Use covered cool-packs.	*Instruct Pam in a home exercise program that includes postural and nerve gliding exercises.*	*Trial a variety of ergonomic equipment options available in the clinic.*	*Set up simulated workspace and identify potential modifications for environment and work habits.*
Issue catalog featuring ergonomic equipment.	*Discuss the purpose and benefit of using the splints and how doing the exercises will positively affect her engagement in occupations.*		
Fit and issue splints for day and night.			
Issue home exercise program.			

Session Plan—Intervention Continuum

Identify one of Pam's priority occupations:

Using interventions from the "Intervention Brainstorm," develop an occupational therapy session for Pam.

Adjunctive Interventions	Enabling Interventions	Purposeful Interventions	Occupation-Based Interventions

Now develop a second occupational therapy session for Pam. Consider progressing to the next session or to a session that is closer to the discontinuation of occupational therapy intervention.

Identify which of Pam's priority occupation(s) will be addressed in this session:

Adjunctive Interventions	Enabling Interventions	Purposeful Interventions	Occupation-Based Interventions

Sample Session Plans

Two sample session plans that may be included in Pam's occupational therapy intervention follow.

Session Plan #1

A Adjunctive Interventions	E Enabling Interventions	P Purposeful Interventions	O Occupation-Based Interventions
Fit and issue splints for day and night.	Instruct Pam in a home exercise program that includes postural and nerve gliding exercises. Discuss the purpose and benefit of using the splints and how doing the exercises will positively affect Pam's engagement in occupations.	Pam trials a variety of ergonomic equipment options available in the clinic.	

Session Plan #2

A Adjunctive Interventions	E Enabling Interventions	P Purposeful Interventions	O Occupation-Based Interventions
Issue a brochure describing pathology and prevention strategies. Use covered cool-packs.			Pam brings her racquetball racquet to therapy for grip and form assessment and recommendations for modifications. Pam sets up simulated workspace and identifies potential modifications for environment and work habits.

Check Your Thinking 7-10

Review the sample sessions and Pam's client-centered interview. Which of Pam's priority occupations do you think the sample sessions address?

Session #1:

```
┌─────────────────────────────────────────────────────────────────────┐
│                                                                       │
│                                                                       │
│                                                                       │
└─────────────────────────────────────────────────────────────────────┘
```

Session #2:

```
┌─────────────────────────────────────────────────────────────────────┐
│                                                                       │
│                                                                       │
│                                                                       │
└─────────────────────────────────────────────────────────────────────┘
```

What If?

Consider how each of the following "what if?" situations would affect your intervention plan for Pam.

1. What if you discovered that Pam's workstation included a stool with no armrests, a traditional phone, and a desk/keyboard height that puts her wrists at 30 degrees of extension?

2. What if Pam's condition was worse at the end of her four occupational therapy sessions?

3. What if Pam's supervisor was not agreeable to having her use ergonomic equipment in the workplace and told her that she would not be paid for any time spent doing her exercises?

4. What if Pam had carpal tunnel release surgery and returned for occupational therapy intervention?

CLINICAL SCENARIO #11—STEPHEN

Setting:	Preschool
Diagnosis:	Down's syndrome
Estimated duration of intervention:	School year
Anticipated discharge plan:	Integrated preschool classroom with learning support

Occupational Profile and Analysis of Occupational Performance

Stephen is the 3-year-old son of Frank and Marion and the brother of 2-year-old Justin. He is in his first year of preschool in a classroom of 12 children, of whom five have special needs. A special education teacher, a full-time paraprofessional, and a full-time occupational therapy assistant staff the classroom.

Stephen is able to follow simple one-step verbal instructions accompanied by gestures and pointing. He is nonverbal and uses a signing system developed by his family that consists of approximately 15 different signs. Stephen's gross motor skills are mildly delayed (less than 25 percent) and he exhibits decreased strength in the proximal musculature of his upper and lower extremities. He is able to kick a ball, ambulate independently on all surfaces, and negotiate steps nonreciprocally. Stephen's fine motor capabilities are consistent with that of an 18-month-old. Stephen's overall muscle tone is low. He has impaired oral motor control, which results in drooling and loss of food and liquids. Stephen is a "picky" eater who self-feeds finger foods but is unable to use utensils independently. He uses a spout cup for liquids. Stephen's attention span for activities that are enjoyable to him is approximately five minutes. He has a significantly lower attention span (15–20 seconds) for undesirable activities. When given a choice, he will choose a gross motor game or activity over one that requires the use of fine motor skills. In addition, Stephen isolates himself and does not easily engage in play activities with his peers. Stephen's parents work opposite shifts so that one of them is able to be at home at all times. Frank and Marion are very supportive, open to suggestions, and have realistic expectations for Stephen's development.

Identification of Strengths and Problems

Make a list of Stephen's strengths and problems based on your review of his occupational profile and analysis of occupational performance.

> **My List of Stephen's Strengths:**

> **My List of Stephen's Problems:**

Identification of Areas of Occupation, Performance Skills, Performance Patterns, and Performance Contexts

Using Appendix F, make a list of the areas of occupation, performance skills, performance patterns, and/or performance contexts that you anticipate addressing in Stephen's occupational therapy intervention plan.

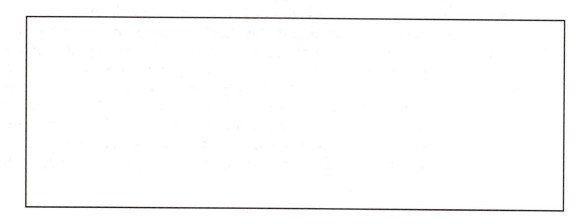

Client-Centered Interview Results

The following is Stephen's client-centered interview, which includes a list of the occupations that his parents and classroom teacher identified as needing, wanting, and expecting Stephen to perform. The occupations Stephen's parents and teacher identified as priority areas for improvement are circled.

Occupations I need to do:

(1.) Use the toilet

2. Eat a variety of foods

(3.) Feed himself with a fork and spoon

(4.) Communicate better with people outside of his immediate family

5. Sit, look, and listen in the classroom

Occupations I want to do:

(1.) Play with his brother

(2.) Play with other children

3. Have better fine motor skills for school

4. Communicate better with the teacher and classmates

Occupations I am expected to do:

1. Effectively communicate his basic needs and wants

2. Play with other children and his brother

(3.) Take his coat on and off

4. Use the toilet

Intervention Brainstorm

Make a list of interventions to include in Stephen's occupational therapy intervention plan based on Stephen's occupational profile and analysis of occupational performance, the strengths and problems you identified, and Stephen's client-centered interview results.

Intervention Continuum

A Adjunctive Interventions	E Enabling Interventions	P Purposeful Interventions	O Occupation-Based Interventions
Interventions that prepare for performance and participation	*Interventions that focus on performance skills*	*Interventions that have a pre-determined goal and facilitate practice and problem solving*	*Interventions that are perceived as desirable, match individualized goals, and occur in appropriate context*

The next step is to categorize the interventions you identified in the Intervention Brainstorm activity according to the intervention continuum. Designate the category into which each intervention falls by labeling the interventions as "A," "E," "P," or "O" to reflect them as adjunctive, enabling, purposeful, or occupation-based.

Sample Intervention Continuum

Sample interventions categorized in the intervention continuum that may be included in Stephen's occupational therapy intervention plan follow.

Adjunctive Interventions	Enabling Interventions	Purposeful Interventions	Occupation-Based Interventions
Provide suggestions to parents for enhancing play skills and opportunities. Reinforcement of picture-based communication system with parents for more universal applicability. Instruct parents/teacher in play and self-care opportunities for enhancing oral motor control.	Weight-bearing activities.	String beads. Snap/unsnap with pop-beads. Stack blocks. Blow through a straw to push a cotton ball across the table to a classmate who will blow it back.	Manage pants for toileting. Manage clothing (e.g., coat, hat, gloves). Use picture-based communication system to identify articles of clothing to therapist. Feed himself cereal with hand-over-hand assistance and drink milk through a straw.

Session Plan—Intervention Continuum

Identify one of Stephen's priority occupations:

Using interventions from the "Intervention Brainstorm," develop an occupational therapy session for Stephen.

Adjunctive Interventions	Enabling Interventions	Purposeful Interventions	Occupation-Based Interventions

Now develop a second occupational therapy session for Stephen. Consider progressing to the next session or to a session that is closer to the discontinuation of occupational therapy intervention.

Identify which of Stephen's priority occupation(s) will be addressed in this session:

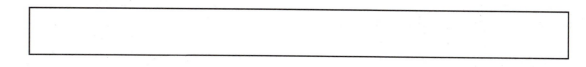

A Adjunctive Interventions	E Enabling Interventions	P Purposeful Interventions	O Occupation-Based Interventions

Sample Session Plans

Two sample session plans that may be included in Stephen's occupational therapy intervention plan follow.

Session Plan #1

A Adjunctive Interventions	E Enabling Interventions	P Purposeful Interventions	O Occupation-Based Interventions
Reinforcement of picture-based communication system with parents for more universal applicability.			*Stephen uses picture-based communication system to identify articles of clothing to therapist.* *Stephen manages clothing (e.g., coat, hat, gloves) upon arrival to and departure from school.*

Session Plan #2

Adjunctive Interventions	Enabling Interventions	Purposeful Interventions	Occupation-Based Interventions
Instruct parents/teacher in play and self-care opportunities for enhancing oral motor control.		*Stephen blows through a straw to push a cotton ball across the table to a classmate who will blow it back to Stephen.*	*Stephen feeds himself cereal with hand-over-hand assistance and drinks his milk through a straw.*

Check Your Thinking 7-11

Review the sample sessions and Stephen's client-centered interview. Which of Stephen's priority occupations do you think the sample sessions address?

Session #1:

Session #2:

What If?

Consider how each of the following "what if?" situations would affect your intervention plan for Stephen.

1. What if there was not an occupational therapy assistant in the classroom on a full-time basis? How would you ensure that your suggestions were being carried out?

2. What if Stephen's parents' goal was for Stephen to "be normal"?

3. What if Stephen's fine motor skills were significantly more developed than his gross motor skills?

4. What if Stephen was the only child with special needs in a typical preschool classroom where the teacher had no experience with special needs children?

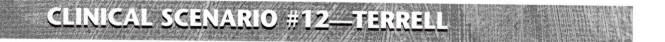

CLINICAL SCENARIO #12—TERRELL

Setting:	In-home services
Diagnoses:	C4–6 diskectomy; previous right hip disarticulation; congestive heart failure
Estimated duration of intervention:	Four weeks
Anticipated discharge plan:	Remain at home

Occupational Profile and Analysis of Occupational Performance

Terrell is a 60-year old male and had surgical removal of a herniated disk followed by six weeks of inpatient rehabilitation. Terrell underwent amputation of his right leg at the hip six years ago as a result of a work-related accident and is on disability. Terrell lives in a first-floor, two-bedroom apartment, with a ramp to enter. The bathroom and kitchen are inaccessible by wheelchair. Terrell lives with his mentally impaired adult daughter, Doris, who requires moderate direction and supervision. Doris completes laundry and light housekeeping, but is unable or unwilling to perform meal preparation, budgeting, or shopping. Prior to his back surgery, Terrell used crutches in the home environment and used a wheelchair for community mobility. He also drove a car, which is a necessity, as he lives in a rural area without public transportation.

Presently, Terrell uses a wheelchair for mobility in the home environment and reports being anxious to "use his crutches again," particularly since he is unable to access the bathroom in the wheelchair. His upper extremity strength is fair bilaterally and he complains of neck and shoulder pain during active end range of motion. Tremors are noted in both arms when Terrell exerts effort (i.e., as he prepares to perform transfers). Terrell requires minimal assistance with bed mobility and moderate to maximal assistance for safety when performing bed, wheelchair, and bedside commode transfers. He has not attempted car transfers because of his strength and endurance limitations. Despite apparent intact cognition, Terrell verbalizes a decreased regard for safety in his efforts to gain independence and reports that he has sustained two falls since returning home.

Identification of Strengths and Problems

Make a list of Terrell's strengths and problems based on your review of his occupational profile and analysis of occupational performance.

My List of Terrell's Strengths:

My List of Terrell's Problems:

Identification of Areas of Occupation, Performance Skills, Performance Patterns, and Performance Contexts

Using Appendix F, make a list of the areas of occupation, performance skills, performance patterns, and/or performance contexts that you anticipate addressing in Terrell's occupational therapy intervention plan.

Client-Centered Interview Results

The following is Terrell's client-centered interview, which includes a list of the occupations that he identified as needing, wanting, and being expected to perform. The occupations Terrell identified as priority areas for improvement are circled.

Occupations I need to do:

1. Get in and out of bed by myself

2. Get in the bathroom and be able to bathe and use the toilet by myself

3. Drive my car

4. Care for my daughter

5. Get out of this wheelchair

Occupations I want to do:

1. Drive my car

2. Take a shower

3. Meet my buddies at the deli

4. Get into the kitchen so I can make our meals

Occupations I am expected to do:

1. Take care of my daughter

2. Take care of myself

Intervention Brainstorm

On the following page, make a list of interventions to include in Terrell's occupational therapy intervention plan based on Terrell's occupational profile and analysis of occupational performance, the strengths and problems you identified, and Terrell's client-centered interview results.

Intervention Continuum

Adjunctive	Enabling	Purposeful	Occupation-Based
Interventions that prepare for performance and participation	Interventions that focus on performance skills	Interventions that have a pre-determined goal and facilitate practice and problem solving	Interventions that are perceived as desirable, match individualized goals, and occur in appropriate context

The next step is to categorize the interventions you identified in the Intervention Brainstorm activity according to the intervention continuum. Designate the category into which each intervention falls by labeling the interventions as "A," "E," "P," or "O" to reflect them as adjunctive, enabling, purposeful, or occupation-based.

Sample Intervention Continuum

Sample interventions categorized in the intervention continuum that may be included in Terrell's occupational therapy intervention plan follow.

A **Adjunctive Interventions**	E **Enabling Interventions**	P **Purposeful Interventions**	O **Occupation-Based Interventions**
Provide recommendations for bathroom safety equipment and information for acquiring items. *Moist heat to decrease joint stiffness and shoulder pain.* *Provide written materials related to home safety and body mechanics.*	*Upper extremity range of motion, strengthening, and weight-bearing exercises.* *Discuss and demonstrate applicability of body mechanics to upper extremity exercise program.* *Discuss and implement safe options for accessing bathroom (wheeled desk chair or stool; removal of door).*	*Practice sit-to-stand transfers from wheelchair using proper body mechanics.* *Access the bathroom and practice tub bench transfers fully clothed.*	*Discuss and facilitate access to community services and programs to improve overall health and well-being (e.g., Meals on Wheels, support programs for daughter, services to aid with home management).* *Practice a car transfer to/from his car with adaptive equipment as needed in the parking lot.* *Observe and assess Terrell's skill as he instructs Doris to set-up bathroom equipment since he does not wish to keep transfer bench in tub when not being used.* *Complete bathing using adaptive equipment in bathroom with supervision and assistance.*

Session Plan—Intervention Continuum

Identify one of Terrell's priority occupations:

Using interventions from the "Intervention Brainstorm," develop an occupational therapy session for Terrell.

A Adjunctive Interventions	**E** Enabling Interventions	**P** Purposeful Interventions	**O** Occupation-Based Interventions

Now develop a second occupational therapy session for Terrell. Consider progressing to the next session or to a session that is closer to the discontinuation of occupational therapy intervention.

Identify which of Terrell's priority occupation(s) will be addressed in this session:

A Adjunctive Interventions	**E** Enabling Interventions	**P** Purposeful Interventions	**O** Occupation-Based Interventions

Sample Session Plans

Two sample session plans that may be included in Terrell's occupational therapy intervention plan follow.

Session Plan #1

A Adjunctive Interventions	E Enabling Interventions	P Purposeful Interventions	O Occupation-Based Interventions
Moist heat to decrease joint stiffness and shoulder pain.	Upper extremity range of motion, strengthening, and weight-bearing exercises.	Terrell practices sit-to-stand transfers from wheelchair using proper body mechanics.	Discuss and facilitate access to community services and programs to improve overall health and well-being (e.g., Meals on Wheels, support programs for daughter, services to aid with home management).

Session Plan #2

A Adjunctive Interventions	E Enabling Interventions	P Purposeful Interventions	O Occupation-Based Interventions
Provide recommendations for bathroom safety equipment and information for acquiring items.	Discuss and implement safe options for accessing bathroom (wheeled desk chair or stool; removal of door).	Terrell accesses the bathroom and practices tub bench transfers fully clothed.	Observe and assess Terrell's skill as he instructs Doris to set-up bathroom equipment since he does not wish to keep transfer bench in tub when not being used.

Check Your Thinking 7-12

Review the sample sessions and Terrell's client-centered interview. Which of Terrell's priority occupations do you think the sample sessions address?

Session #1:

Session #2:

What If?

Consider how each of the following "what if?" situations would affect your intervention plan for Terrell.

1. What if Terrell's daughter was 8-years-old?

2. What if Terrell's upper extremity weakness did not improve?

3. What if Terrell was noncompliant with his exercise program?

4. What if Terrell was a cashier at a convenience store?

CLINICAL SCENARIO #13—TRUDY

Setting:	Community needle exchange drop-in center
Diagnoses:	Polysubstance dependence; major depressive disorder
Estimated duration of intervention:	Two to three sessions per week; services are open-ended; discharge is to be determined by Trudy
Anticipated discharge plan:	Remain at the women's shelter with goal to establish residence in a studio apartment

Occupational Profile and Analysis of Occupational Performance

Trudy is an unemployed, homeless 31-year-old female who has been attending groups for two weeks. For the past seven years, Trudy has been actively using a variety of drugs and has not been involved in a drug treatment program. Trudy graduated from college with a degree in criminal studies. She hopes to attend law school and become a trial attorney. Trudy described her adolescence as participating in soccer and the debate team, being class representative to the student council, having a large circle of friends, and doing needlecraft as a hobby. It was during college that Trudy first began to experiment with drugs. She maintained this routine after college graduation and while working as an administrative assistant at a prestigious law firm. She began getting high every day and initially was able to maintain her performance at work and home. However, her work performance began to decrease and she was placed on probation. She was finally terminated one year ago due to her poor performance, appearance, and attendance.

Trudy has multiple soft tissue injuries and an untreated fracture of her right ulna, which she will not discuss. She exhibits active range of motion restrictions of her right forearm and wrist as well as difficulty manipulating small objects with her right hand. Last week, during a routine visit to the drop-in center, she requested an HIV test. She is waiting for the results of this test. Trudy's appearance is disheveled and she is often unclean. She does try to bathe at the sink in the bathroom at the center. Her nutritional intake is poor and her dental hygiene appears limited as noted by missing teeth and odor. Trudy is unable to concentrate for longer than seven minutes on any given activity. She exhibits ineffective problem-solving ability and, when presented with an obstacle, will typically walk away to avoid the problem. Trudy rarely initiates conversation with others. She reports feelings of hopelessness and past suicidal ideation.

Identification of Strengths and Problems

Make a list of Trudy's strengths and problems based on your review of her occupational profile and analysis of occupational performance.

My List of Trudy's Strengths:

My List of Trudy's Problems:

Identification of Areas of Occupation, Performance Skills, Performance Patterns, and Performance Contexts

Using Appendix F, make a list of the areas of occupation, performance skills, performance patterns, and/or performance contexts that you anticipate addressing in Trudy's occupational therapy intervention plan.

Client-Centered Interview Results

The following is Trudy's client-centered interview, which includes a list of the occupations that she identified as needing, wanting, and being expected to perform. The occupations Trudy identified as priority areas for improvement are circled.

Occupations I need to do:

①. Get a job

2. Be healthy

3. Take better care of myself

④. Get my right arm moving better

Occupations I want to do:

①. Get an apartment

②. Be a healthier person

3. Have a healthy relationship with a partner

4. Become a wife and have children

5. Have a relationship with my sister

Occupations I am expected to do:

1. Work

2. Get off the streets

3. Be healthier

4. Be clean

5. Dress better

Intervention Brainstorm

Make a list of interventions to include in Trudy's occupational therapy intervention plan based on Trudy's occupational profile and analysis of occupational performance, the strengths and problems you identified, and Trudy's client-centered interview results.

Intervention Continuum

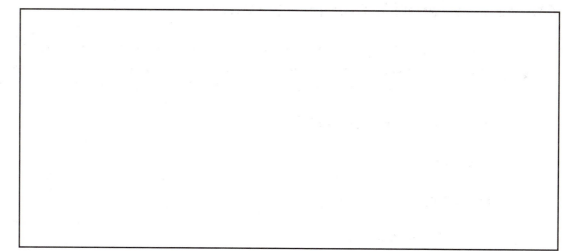

Adjunctive Interventions	Enabling Interventions	Purposeful Interventions	Occupation-Based Interventions
Interventions that prepare for performance and participation	*Interventions that focus on performance skills*	*Interventions that have a pre-determined goal and facilitate practice and problem solving*	*Interventions that are perceived as desirable, match individualized goals, and occur in appropriate context*

The next step is to categorize the interventions you identified in the Intervention Brainstorm activity according to the intervention continuum. Designate the category into which each intervention falls by labeling the interventions as "A," "E," "P," or "O" to reflect them as adjunctive, enabling, purposeful, or occupation-based.

Sample Intervention Continuum

Sample interventions categorized in the intervention continuum that may be included in Trudy's occupational therapy intervention plan follow.

A Adjunctive Interventions	**E** Enabling Interventions	**P** Purposeful Interventions	**O** Occupation-Based Interventions
Issue handout for right upper extremity active range of motion and coordination exercises. *Provide basic information on health and wellness (i.e., nutrition, personal safety, etc.).*	*Instruction in and repeat demonstration of right upper extremity active range of motion and coordination exercises.* *Discuss job interview skills (e.g., arriving on time, appropriate dress, responding to and asking questions appropriately).* *Review and complete sample job applications.*	*Role-play assertive communication and interviewing for employment positions and receive peer feedback.* *Complete craft activities of graded complexity and duration to improve fine motor coordination and concentration levels.* *Develop healthy meal menus.*	*Use a journal or other mechanism to record her decisions, actions, and the outcomes.* *Participate in former leisure interests (i.e., needlecraft).* *Plan grocery shopping for food needed to prepare a healthy meal menu; follow through with shopping outside of session; process performance during next session.* *Identify potential employment opportunities through the newspaper and other means.*

Session Plan—Intervention Continuum

Identify one of Trudy's priority occupations:

Using interventions from the "Intervention Brainstorm," develop an occupational therapy session for Trudy.

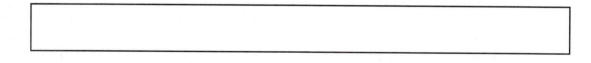 Adjunctive Interventions	Enabling Interventions	Purposeful Interventions	Occupation-Based Interventions

Now develop a second occupational therapy session for Trudy. Consider progressing to the next session or to a session that is closer to the discontinuation of occupational therapy intervention.

Identify which of Trudy's priority occupation(s) will be addressed in this session:

Adjunctive Interventions	Enabling Interventions	Purposeful Interventions	Occupation-Based Interventions

Sample Session Plans

Two sample session plans that may be included in Trudy's occupational therapy intervention follow.

Session Plan #1

Adjunctive Interventions	**Enabling Interventions**	**Purposeful Interventions**	**Occupation-Based Interventions**
Issue handout for right upper extremity active range of motion and coordination exercises.	Instruction in and repeat demonstration of right upper extremity active range of motion and coordination exercises.	Trudy participates in craft activities of graded complexity and duration to improve fine motor coordination and concentration levels.	

Session Plan #2

Adjunctive Interventions	**Enabling Interventions**	**Purposeful Interventions**	**Occupation-Based Interventions**
	Review and complete sample job applications. Discuss job interview skills.	Trudy role-plays interviewing for employment positions and receives peer feedback.	Trudy identifies potential employment opportunities through the newspaper and other means.

Check Your Thinking 7-13

Review the sample sessions and Trudy's client-centered interview. Which of Trudy's priority occupations do you think the sample sessions address?

Session #1:

Session #2:

```
┌─────────────────────────────────────────────────────────────────┐
│                                                                   │
│                                                                   │
│                                                                   │
│                                                                   │
└─────────────────────────────────────────────────────────────────┘
```

What If?

Consider how each of the following "what if?" situations would affect your intervention plan for Trudy.

1. What if Trudy's appearance began to worsen and she lost weight?

2. What if Trudy's level of concentration did not improve?

3. What if Trudy verbalized suicidal ideation during a session?

4. What if Trudy had poor insight into her capabilities and skill performance and wanted to pursue a job for which she was unqualified?

CLINICAL SCENARIO #14—WALTER

Setting:	Acute care hospital
Diagnosis:	Schizophrenia
Estimated duration of intervention:	Two weeks
Anticipated discharge plan:	Unknown

Occupational Profile and Analysis of Occupational Performance

Walter is a 28-year-old male who lives with his younger brother, Scott, in Scott's apartment. Walter has a history of multiple psychiatric hospitalizations beginning at the age of 19. He currently works part-time at a local grocery store where he primarily stocks shelves and retrieves carts. Walter has been working at this particular job for four months. He has never held a job for longer than nine months. He is currently suspended due to absenteeism, becoming argumentative with customers and other employees, and for not meeting the grooming and dress standards. Scott reported that Walter's behavior has deteriorated over the last three weeks and he suspects that Walter has stopped taking his medication. Scott said that Walter barricaded himself in his room and police assistance was required to transport him to the hospital. Scott expressed that he may not want Walter to live with him after this hospitalization.

Walter's affect is flat. His speech is slow and disorganized with loose associations. His appearance is unkempt with dirty, layered clothing, unclean hair, and notable body odor. Walter requires step-by-step instruction and demonstration to complete even simple tasks. He appears to be responding to auditory hallucinations. He makes minimal eye contact and seems somewhat anxious, especially in open areas with increased activity and people. His strength, coordination, and endurance are limited. Walter also presents with a closed posture and rocks his body back and forth slightly when sitting. He is able to complete basic self-care tasks; however, he requires supervision and verbal cues to perform tasks safely and adequately.

Identification of Strengths and Problems

Make a list of Walter's strengths and problems based on your review of his occupational profile and analysis of occupational performance.

```
┌─────────────────────────────────────────────────────────────────────┐
│ My List of Walter's Strengths:                                        │
│                                                                       │
│                                                                       │
│                                                                       │
│                                                                       │
│                                                                       │
└─────────────────────────────────────────────────────────────────────┘
```

```
┌─────────────────────────────────────────────────────────────────────┐
│ My List of Walter's Problems:                                         │
│                                                                       │
│                                                                       │
│                                                                       │
│                                                                       │
└─────────────────────────────────────────────────────────────────────┘
```

Identification of Areas of Occupation, Performance Skills, Performance Patterns, and Performance Contexts

Using Appendix F, make a list of the areas of occupation, performance skills, performance patterns, and/or performance contexts that you anticipate addressing in Walter's occupational therapy intervention plan.

Client-Centered Interview Results

The following is Walter's client-centered interview, which includes a list of the occupations that his brother, Scott, identified as needing, wanting, and expecting Walter to perform as Walter was unable to provide appropriate information. The occupations Scott identified as priority areas for improvement are circled.

Occupations I need to do:

1. Walter needs to take his medications

2. Bathe and dress himself

3. Clean his room

4. Go to work

5. Help around the apartment (e.g., meal preparation, housekeeping)

Occupations I want to do:

1. Walter likes to listen to music

2. Walter likes to sleep

3. Walter wants to work

4. Walter wants to live in his own apartment

Occupations I am expected to do:

1. Take his medications

2. Bathe and dress himself

3. Pay his share of the expenses

4. Go to work

5. Help clean the apartment

Intervention Brainstorm

Make a list of interventions to include in Walter's occupational therapy intervention plan based on Walter's occupational profile and analysis of occupational performance, the strengths and problems you identified, and Walter's client-centered interview results.

Intervention Continuum

Adjunctive	**Enabling**	**Purposeful**	**Occupation-Based**
Interventions that prepare for performance and participation	*Interventions that focus on performance skills*	*Interventions that have a pre-determined goal and facilitate practice and problem solving*	*Interventions that are perceived as desirable, match individualized goals, and occur in appropriate context*

The next step is to categorize the interventions you identified in the Intervention Brainstorm activity according to the intervention continuum. Designate the category into which each intervention falls by labeling the interventions as "A," "E," "P," or "O" to reflect them as adjunctive, enabling, purposeful, or occupation-based.

Sample Intervention Continuum

Sample interventions categorized in the intervention continuum that may be included in Walter's occupational therapy intervention plan follow.

A Adjunctive Interventions	E Enabling Interventions	P Purposeful Interventions	O Occupation-Based Interventions
Provide educational information (e.g., diagnosis, medication, community resources) to Walter and Scott.	Movement group.	Grooming tasks in the OT clinic. Graded craft activities. Cooking group (set-up, cooking steps, clean-up). Money management activities. Medication management activities. Simulate Walter's work-related activities.	Morning self-care tasks in his room with supervision and assistance as needed. Light housekeeping tasks in his room (making bed, wiping sink area, tidying desk area and closet). Washes and dries his laundry using unit facilities. With guidance, Walter and Scott create a list of household expectations for themselves and consequences if expectations are not met.

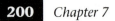

Session Plan—Intervention Continuum

Identify one of Walter's priority occupations:

Using interventions from the "Intervention Brainstorm," develop an occupational therapy session for Walter.

A Adjunctive Interventions	**E** Enabling Interventions	**P** Purposeful Interventions	**O** Occupation-Based Interventions

Now develop a second occupational therapy session for Walter. Consider progressing to the next session or to a session that is closer to the discontinuation of occupational therapy intervention.

Identify which of Walter's priority occupation(s) will be addressed in this session:

A Adjunctive Interventions	**E** Enabling Interventions	**P** Purposeful Interventions	**O** Occupation-Based Interventions

Sample Session Plans

Two sample session plans that may be included in Walter's occupational therapy intervention follow.

Session Plan #1

A Adjunctive Interventions	**E** Enabling Interventions	**P** Purposeful Interventions	**O** Occupation-Based Interventions
			Walter completes morning self-care tasks in his room with supervision and assistance as needed. *Walter performs light housekeeping tasks in his room (making bed, wiping sink area, tidying desk area and closet).*

Session Plan #2

A Adjunctive Interventions	**E** Enabling Interventions	**P** Purposeful Interventions	**O** Occupation-Based Interventions
		Walter participates in cooking group (set-up, cooking steps, clean-up)	

Check Your Thinking 7-14

Review the sample sessions and Walter's client-centered interview. Which of Walter's priority occupations do you think the sample sessions address?

Session #1:

```



```

Session #2:

```



```

What If?

Consider how each of the following "what if?" situations would affect your intervention plan for Walter.

1. What if Walter's anticipated discharge plan is to reside at a long-term structured residential facility?

2. What if Walter's employer terminates him?

3. What if Walter became aggressive during a therapy session?

4. What if Walter experiences delusional behavior (e.g., his brother and coworkers are trying to poison him; his boss is from an alien planet)?

APPENDIX A

Activities of Daily Living (ADL)

- Bathing, showering
- Bowel and bladder management
- Dressing
- Eating
- Feeding
- Functional mobility
- Personal device care
- Personal hygiene and grooming
- Sexual activity
- Sleep/rest
- Toilet hygiene

Instrumental Activities of Daily Living (IADL)

- Care of others
- Care of pets
- Communication device use
- Community mobility
- Financial management
- Health management and maintenance
- Home establishment and management
- Meal preparation and clean-up
- Safety procedures and emergency responses
- Shopping

Education

➤ Formal educational participation

➤ Exploration of informal personal educational needs or interests

➤ Informal personal education participation

Work

➤ Employment interests and pursuits

➤ Employment seeking and acquisition

➤ Job performance

➤ Retirement preparation and adjustment

➤ Volunteer exploration

➤ Volunteer participation

Play

➤ Play exploration

➤ Play participation

Leisure

➤ Leisure exploration

➤ Leisure participation

Social Participation

➤ Community

➤ Family

➤ Peer, friend

NOTE: From "Occupational therapy practice framework: Domain and process" by the American Occupational Therapy Association, 2002, *American Journal of Occupational Therapy, 56,* 620–621. Copyright 2002 by the American Occupational Therapy Association, Inc. Adapted with permission.

References

American Occupational Therapy Association. (1994). Uniform terminology for occupational therapy—third edition. *American Journal of Occupational Therapy, 48,* 1047–1054.

American Occupational Therapy Association. (2002). Occupational therapy practice framework: Domain and process. *American Journal of Occupational Therapy, 56,* 609–639.

CHECK YOUR THINKING ANSWERS

If your response differs from the answer provided, review the description of the intervention continuum category. Assigning an intervention to a category is influenced by the level of familiarity with the intervention and considerations related to specific client populations and/or practice settings, so answers may vary.

Answers to Check Your Thinking 3-2

_____	dowel rod exercises
A	scar massage
_____	pulling small pegs out of putty
A	hot or ice pack
_____	placing pegs in a peg board
A	issuing a handout listing stress management strategies
A	paraffin wax dips
_____	upper extremity exercises with a resistive band
A	compression wrap to decrease edema
_____	baking cookies in the occupational therapy kitchen
_____	handwriting exercises
A	providing a letter strip for student's desk
_____	stacking cones
_____	bean bag toss game
A	issuing adaptive equipment

_____	loading dishes in the occupational therapy department dishwasher
A	fabricating and fitting a splint
A	providing teachers with information related to sensory integration techniques
A	wheelchair positioning techniques
_____	shoulder range of motion arc
A	written information for caregivers
_____	discussion of relaxation techniques and brainstorming of potential applications
_____	locating and removing items from a rice bin
_____	stringing beads to make a necklace
_____	finger ladder
_____	styling hair with own supplies
_____	folding towels that belong to the occupational therapy clinic
_____	copying a paragraph from a magazine
_____	safety obstacle course
_____	cleaning the mirror in the occupational therapy bathroom

Answers to Check Your Thinking 3-5

E	dowel rod exercises
_____	scar massage
E	pulling small pegs out of putty
_____	hot or ice pack
E	placing pegs in a peg board
_____	issuing a handout listing stress management strategies
_____	paraffin wax dips
E	upper extremity exercises with a resistive band
_____	compression wrap to decrease edema
_____	baking cookies in the occupational therapy kitchen
E	handwriting exercises
_____	providing a letter strip for student's desk

E   stacking cones

_____   bean bag toss game

_____   issuing adaptive equipment

_____   loading dishes in the occupational therapy department dishwasher

_____   fabricating and fitting a splint

_____   providing teachers with information related to sensory integration techniques

_____   wheelchair positioning techniques

E   shoulder range of motion arc

_____   written information for caregivers

E   discussion of relaxation techniques and brainstorming of potential applications

E   locating and removing items from a rice bin

_____   stringing beads to make a necklace

E   finger ladder

_____   styling hair with own supplies

_____   folding towels that belong to the occupational therapy clinic

_____   copying a paragraph from a magazine

_____   safety obstacle course

_____   cleaning the mirror in the occupational therapy bathroom

Answers to Check Your Thinking 3-8

_____   dowel rod exercises

_____   scar massage

_____   pulling small pegs out of putty

_____   hot or ice pack

_____   placing pegs in a peg board

_____   issuing a handout listing stress management strategies

_____   paraffin wax dips

_____   upper extremity exercises with a resistive band

_____   compression wrap to decrease edema

P	baking cookies in the occupational therapy kitchen
_____	handwriting exercises
_____	providing a letter strip for student's desk
_____	stacking cones
P	bean bag toss game
_____	issuing adaptive equipment
P	loading dishes in the occupational therapy department dishwasher
_____	fabricating and fitting a splint
_____	providing teachers with information related to sensory integration techniques
_____	wheelchair positioning techniques
_____	shoulder range of motion arc
_____	written information for caregivers
_____	discussion of relaxation techniques and brainstorming of potential applications
_____	locating and removing items from a rice bin
P	stringing beads to make a necklace
_____	finger ladder
_____	styling hair with own supplies
P	folding towels that belong to the occupational therapy clinic
P	copying a paragraph from a magazine
P	safety obstacle course
P	cleaning the mirror in the occupational therapy bathroom

Answers to Check Your Thinking 3-11

_____	lifting a crate that weighs as much as his child
O	completing grooming while standing at the sink
O	making dinner for his wife
_____	placing pegs in a peg board
_____	completing upper extremity exercise for affected arm
O	transcribing class notes on a chalkboard

O   transferring in and out of own car in facility parking lot

_____   folding towels that belong to the occupational therapy department

_____   contrast bath

_____   copy a recipe for beef although he dislikes meat

O   dribbling a basketball on the facility basketball court

O   preparing his child's favorite lunch meal

O   preparing notes from biology book

_____   pulling small pegs out of putty

_____   standing in a standing box to increase standing endurance

Answers to Check Your Thinking 3-13

P   lifting and carrying a grocery bag filled with occupational therapy clinic food items

A   fluidotherapy

P   making chocolate chip cookies in occupational therapy clinic to share with staff and other clients

E   placing clothespins on a rod

E   pinch exercises with putty

O   copying a recipe for a friend

O   telephoning a grandchild

P   cutting out coupons collected by the occupational therapy staff

P   bowling in the clinic

O   completing self-care tasks in the morning with own adaptive equipment

P   watering plants in the occupational therapy clinic

P   making a macramé plant hanger

O   finishing own latch-hook project brought to the clinic by a family member

E   transferring from wheelchair to the mat table

O   purchasing a card for a friend at the gift shop

P   brushing teeth in the occupational therapy clinic

E   upper extremity skateboard

P	reading a self-chosen magazine article when standing at table edge
P	role-playing a scenario dealing with anger and management techniques
P	completing a sample check-writing task
P	following a functional ambulation clinic obstacle course with walker
O	hanging cards received from friends and family in the hospital room with a reacher
A	verbal education on how to use a reacher
E	repeated retrieval of objects from the floor using a reacher
A	wearing a resting hand splint during sleeping hours
O	use of adaptive equipment when eating breakfast

APPENDIX C

STEP 1: Consider your primary practice setting when responding to the following questions.

What is your occupational therapy practice setting (i.e., acute care, rehabilitation, school system, long-term care, home health, outpatient, etc.)?

What are the typical diagnoses or conditions of your clients?

What is the gender distribution of your clients?

_____ % female

_____ % male

What is the age distribution of your clients?

_____ % birth–3 years

_____ % 4–9 years

_____ % 10–15 years

_____ % 16–21 years

_____ % 22–40 years

_____ % 41–65 years

_____ % 66–80 years

_____ % 80+ years

What are the typical occupational roles of your clients?

```
┌─────────────────────────────────────────────────────────┐
│                                                           │
│                                                           │
└─────────────────────────────────────────────────────────┘
```

What is the average frequency that your clients receive occupational therapy services?

_____ daily

_____ twice daily

_____ # of sessions

_____ other—describe:

What is the average duration that your clients receive occupational therapy services?

_____ 1 week or less

_____ 2–3 weeks

_____ 4–6 weeks

_____ > 6 weeks

_____ other—describe:

What is the typical discharge destination of your clients?

```
┌─────────────────────────────────────────────────────────┐
│                                                           │
│                                                           │
└─────────────────────────────────────────────────────────┘
```

What are the common reimbursement sources for your occupational therapy services?

```
┌─────────────────────────────────────────────────────────┐
│                                                           │
│                                                           │
└─────────────────────────────────────────────────────────┘
```

STEP 2: Consider the practice setting and clients you described in Step 1. As you review the occupations, skills, patterns, and contexts in Table C-1, put a check mark to the left of the items that are typical problem areas for your clients.

Table C-1   Areas of Occupation, Performance Skills, Performance Patterns, and Performance Contexts.

✔	AREAS OF OCCUPATION	INTERVENTION	A	E	P	O
	Activities of Daily Living					
	Bathing, showering					
	Bowel and bladder management					
	Dressing					
	Eating					
	Feeding					

| Table C-1 | Areas of Occupation, Performance Skills, Performance Patterns, and Performance Contexts. *(continued)* |

✔	AREAS OF OCCUPATION	INTERVENTION	A	E	P	O
	Functional mobility					
	Personal device care					
	Personal hygiene and grooming					
	Sexual activity					
	Sleep/rest					
	Toilet hygiene					
	Instrumental Activities of Daily Living					
	Care of others					
	Care of pets					
	Communication device use					
	Community mobility					
	Financial management					
	Health management and maintenance					
	Home establishment and management					
	Meal preparation and clean-up					
	Safety procedures and emergency responses					
	Shopping					
	Education					
	Formal educational participation					
	Exploration of informal personal educational needs or interests					
	Informal personal education participation					
	Work					
	Employment interests and pursuits					

(continues)

Table C-1	Areas of Occupation, Performance Skills, Performance Patterns, and Performance Contexts. *(continued)*				
✔ **AREAS OF OCCUPATION**	**INTERVENTION**	**A**	**E**	**P**	**O**
Employment seeking and acquisition					
Job performance					
Retirement preparation and adjustment					
Volunteer exploration					
Volunteer participation					
Play					
Play exploration					
Play participation					
Leisure					
Leisure exploration					
Leisure participation					
Social participation					
Community					
Family					
Peer, friend					
✔ **PERFORMANCE SKILLS**	**INTERVENTION**	**A**	**E**	**P**	**O**
Sensorimotor					
Sensory awareness					
Sensory processing					
Tactile					
Proprioceptive					
Vestibular					
Visual					
Auditory					
Gustatory					
Olfactory					
Perceptual processing					
Stereognosis					
Kinesthesia					
Pain response					

Table C-1	Areas of Occupation, Performance Skills, Performance Patterns, and Performance Contexts. *(continued)*				
✔ **PERFORMANCE SKILLS**	**INTERVENTION**	**A**	**E**	**P**	**O**
Body scheme					
Right/left discrimination					
Form constancy					
Position in space					
Visual-closure					
Figure ground					
Depth perception					
Spatial relations					
Topographical orientation					
Neuromusculoskeletal					
Reflexes					
Range of motion					
Muscle tone					
Strength					
Endurance					
Postural control					
Postural alignment					
Soft tissue integrity					
Motor skills					
Gross coordination					
Crossing the midline					
Laterality					
Bilateral integration					
Motor control					
Praxis					
Fine coordination					
Visual-motor integration					
Oral-motor control					
Cognition					
Level of arousal					

(continues)

Table C-1 Areas of Occupation, Performance Skills, Performance Patterns, and Performance Contexts. *(continued)*

✔	PERFORMANCE SKILLS	INTERVENTION	A	E	P	O
	Orientation					
	Recognition					
	Attention span					
	Initiation of activity					
	Termination of activity					
	Memory					
	Sequencing					
	Categorization					
	Concept formation					
	Spatial operations					
	Problem solving					
	Learning					
	Generalization					
	Psychosocial/Psychological					
	Psychological					
	Values					
	Interests					
	Self-concept					
	Social					
	Role performance					
	Social conduct					
	Interpersonal skills					
	Self-expression					
	Self-management					
	Coping skills					
	Time management					
	Self-control					
✔	PERFORMANCE PATTERNS	INTERVENTION	A	E	P	O
	Habits					
	Routines					
	Roles					

Table C-1	Areas of Occupation, Performance Skills, Performance Patterns, and Performance Contexts. (continued)				
✔ **PERFORMANCE CONTEXTS**	**INTERVENTION**	**A**	**E**	**P**	**O**
Cultural					
Physical					
Social					
Personal					
Spiritual					
Temporal					
Virtual					

Note: The areas of occupation, performance patterns, and performance contexts sections are from "Occupational therapy practice framework: Domain and process" by the American Occupational Therapy Association, 2002, *American Journal of Occupational Therapy, 56,* 620–623. Copyright 2002 by the American Occupational Therapy Association, Inc. Adapted with permission. The performance skills section is from the rescinded "Uniform terminology for occupational therapy—third edition" by the American Occupational Therapy Association, 1994, *American Journal of Occupational Therapy, 48,* 1047–1054. Copyright 1994 by the American Occupational Therapy Association, Inc. Adapted with permission.

STEP 3: Consider the practice setting and clients you described in Step 1. Return to Table C-1 and identify an example(s) of an intervention that you typically use to address the problem occupation, skill, pattern, or context you checked. Write your example(s) in the "Intervention" column.

STEP 4: Return to the interventions you wrote in Table C-1. As you review each intervention try to recall a "real life" clinical situation when you used the intervention with one of your clients. Place a check mark in the box to the right of your intervention that you feel best represents the category of the intervention as reflected in the "real life" example (A = adjunctive interventions; E = enabling interventions; P = purposeful interventions; and O = occupation-based interventions).

STEP 5: Referring back to Table C-1, identify a common area of occupation, performance skill, performance pattern, or performance context that you typically address in your clients' therapy programs. Consider the interventions that you use or could use to address the occupation, skill, pattern, and/or context problems across the continuum categories. Boxes C-1 through C-4 provide you with the opportunity to complete this exercise for a range of occupations, performance skills, performance patterns, and performance contexts.

BOX C-1   Intervention Exercise: Areas of Occupation

	EXAMPLES			
Areas of Occupation	**A** **Adjunctive Interventions**	**E** **Enabling Interventions**	**P** **Purposeful Interventions**	**O** **Occupation-Based Interventions**

BOX C-2   Intervention Exercise: Performance Skills

	EXAMPLES			
Performance Skills	**A** **Adjunctive Interventions**	**E** **Enabling Interventions**	**P** **Purposeful Interventions**	**O** **Occupation-Based Interventions**

BOX C-3   Intervention Exercise: Performance Patterns

	EXAMPLES			
Performance Patterns	**A** **Adjunctive Interventions**	**E** **Enabling Interventions**	**P** **Purposeful Interventions**	**O** **Occupation-Based Interventions**

BOX C-4   Intervention Exercise: Performance Contexts

	EXAMPLES			
Performance Contexts	**A** **Adjunctive Interventions**	**E** **Enabling Interventions**	**P** **Purposeful Interventions**	**O** **Occupation-Based Interventions**

STEP 6:   What circumstances or issues facilitate your ability to include occupation-based interventions in your clients' therapy programs?

What circumstances or issues limit your ability to use occupation-based interventions in your clinical practice?

My wish list: (if you had these things, you would be able to provide occupation-based interventions more consistently.)

References

American Occupational Therapy Association. (1994). Uniform terminology for occupational therapy—third edition. *American Journal of Occupational Therapy, 48,* 1047–1054.

American Occupational Therapy Association. (2002). Occupational therapy practice framework: Domain and process. *American Journal of Occupational Therapy, 56,* 609–639.

APPENDIX D

GROUP INTERVENTION TEMPLATE

Name of group:

Group topic:

Purpose:

Goals of the intervention:

Inclusion criteria for participating in the group:

Conditions/criteria that are contraindicated for participating in the group:

List and describe the specific tasks:

Materials, supplies, and equipment needed:

Time of day restrictions for conducting the group:

Duration of the group:

Location, space, and environmental considerations required for the group:

Leader responsibilities of the group intervention:

Other related information:

APPENDIX E

CATEGORIZING INTERVENTIONS USING THE INTERVENTION CONTINUUM

Intervention Category Key

A	=	Adjunctive intervention
E	=	Enabling intervention
P	=	Purposeful intervention
O	=	Occupation-based intervention

STUDY	PURPOSE OF STUDY	POPULATION	INTERVENTIONS	INTERVENTION CATEGORY

STUDY	PURPOSE OF STUDY	POPULATION	INTERVENTIONS	INTERVENTION CATEGORY

APPENDIX F

AREAS OF OCCUPATION, PERFORMANCE SKILLS, PERFORMANCE PATTERNS, AND PERFORMANCE CONTEXTS

Areas of Occupation

➤ Activities of Daily Living
- Bathing, showering
- Bowel and bladder management
- Dressing
- Eating
- Feeding
- Functional mobility
- Personal device care
- Personal hygiene and grooming
- Sexual activity
- Sleep/rest
- Toilet hygiene

➤ Instrumental Activities of Daily Living
- Care of others
- Care of pets
- Communication device use
- Community mobility
- Financial management
- Health management and maintenance
- Home establishment and management
- Meal preparation and clean-up
- Safety procedures and emergency responses
- Shopping

➤ Education
- Formal educational participation
- Exploration of informal personal educational needs or interests
- Informal personal education participation

➤ Work
- Employment interests and pursuits
- Employment seeking and acquisition
- Job performance
- Retirement preparation and adjustment
- Volunteer exploration
- Volunteer participation

➤ Play
- Play exploration
- Play participation

➤ Leisure
- Leisure exploration
- Leisure participation

➤ Social Participation
- Community
- Family
- Peer, friend

Performance Skills

➤ Sensorimotor
- Sensory awareness
- Sensory processing
  - Tactile
  - Proprioceptive
  - Vestibular
  - Visual
  - Auditory
  - Gustatory
  - Olfactory
- Perceptual processing
  - Stereognosis
  - Kinesthesia
  - Pain response
  - Body scheme

- Right/left discrimination
- Form constancy
- Position in space
- Visual-closure
- Figure ground
- Depth perception
- Spatial relations
- Topographical orientation

➤ Neuromusculoskeletal
- Reflexes
- Range of motion
- Muscle tone
- Strength
- Endurance
- Postural control
- Postural alignment
- Soft tissue integrity

➤ Motor Skills
- Gross coordination
- Crossing the midline
- Laterality
- Bilateral integration
- Motor control
- Praxis
- Fine coordination
- Visual-motor integration
- Oral-motor control

➤ Cognition
- Level of arousal
- Orientation
- Recognition
- Attention span
- Initiation of activity
- Termination of activity
- Memory
- Sequencing
- Categorization

- Concept formation
- Spatial operations
- Problem solving
- Learning
- Generalization

➤ Psychosocial/psychological

- Psychological
  - Values
  - Interests
  - Self-concept
- Social
  - Role performance
  - Social conduct
  - Interpersonal skills
  - Self-expression
- Self-management
  - Coping skills
  - Time management
  - Self-control

Performance patterns

➤ Habits

➤ Routines

➤ Roles

Performance contexts

➤ Cultural

➤ Physical

➤ Social

➤ Personal

➤ Spiritual

➤ Temporal

➤ Virtual

NOTE: The areas of occupation, performance patterns, and performance contexts sections are from "Occupational therapy practice framework: Domain and process" by the American Occupational Therapy Association, 2002, *American Journal of Occupational Therapy, 56,* 609–639. Copyright 2002 by the American Occupational Therapy Association, Inc. Reprinted with permission. The performance skills section is from the rescinded "Uniform terminology for occupational therapy—third edition" by the American Occupational Therapy Association, 1994, *American Journal of Occupational Therapy, 48,* 1055–1059. Copyright 1994 by the American Occupational Therapy Association, Inc. Reprinted with permission.

- Right/left discrimination
- Form constancy
- Position in space
- Visual-closure
- Figure ground
- Depth perception
- Spatial relations
- Topographical orientation

➤ Neuromusculoskeletal
- Reflexes
- Range of motion
- Muscle tone
- Strength
- Endurance
- Postural control
- Postural alignment
- Soft tissue integrity

➤ Motor Skills
- Gross coordination
- Crossing the midline
- Laterality
- Bilateral integration
- Motor control
- Praxis
- Fine coordination
- Visual-motor integration
- Oral-motor control

➤ Cognition
- Level of arousal
- Orientation
- Recognition
- Attention span
- Initiation of activity
- Termination of activity
- Memory
- Sequencing
- Categorization

- Concept formation
- Spatial operations
- Problem solving
- Learning
- Generalization
➤ Psychosocial/psychological
  - Psychological
    - Values
    - Interests
    - Self-concept
  - Social
    - Role performance
    - Social conduct
    - Interpersonal skills
    - Self-expression
  - Self-management
    - Coping skills
    - Time management
    - Self-control

Performance patterns

➤ Habits
➤ Routines
➤ Roles

Performance contexts

➤ Cultural
➤ Physical
➤ Social
➤ Personal
➤ Spiritual
➤ Temporal
➤ Virtual

References

American Occupational Therapy Association. (1994). Uniform terminology for occupational therapy—third edition. *American Journal of Occupational Therapy, 48,* 1047–1054.

American Occupational Therapy Association. (2002). Occupational therapy practice framework: Domain and process. *American Journal of Occupational Therapy, 56,* 609–639.

References

American Occupational Therapy Association. (1994). Uniform terminology for occupational therapy—third edition. *American Journal of Occupational Therapy, 48,* 1047–1054.

American Occupational Therapy Association. (2002). Occupational therapy practice framework: Domain and process. *American Journal of Occupational Therapy, 56,* 609–639.

APPENDIX G

Put *your* client's name and related information in the blank spaces.

Name: _____

Setting: _____

Diagnosis(es): _____

Estimated duration of intervention: _____

Anticipated discharge plan: _____

Occupational Profile and Analysis of Occupational Performance

Identification of Strengths and Problems

List *your* client's strengths and problems based on your review of his or her occupational profile and analysis of occupational performance.

Strengths:

Problems:

Identification of Areas of Occupation, Performance Skills, Performance Patterns, and Performance Contexts

Using Appendix F, make a list of the areas of occupation, performance skills, performance patterns, and/or performance contexts that you anticipate addressing in *your* client's occupational therapy intervention plan.

Client-Centered Interview Results

STEP 1: Ask *your* client to think about the occupations he or she performs during a typical day and provide three to five responses to the following:

Occupations client needs to do:

1.

2.

3.

4.

5.

Occupations client wants to do:

1.

2.

3.

4.

5.

Occupations client is expected to do:

1.

2.

3.

4.

5.

STEP 2: Ask *your* client to circle his or her five most important occupations.

Intervention Brainstorm

Make a list of interventions to include in *your* client's occupational therapy intervention plan based on his or her occupational profile and analysis of occupational performance, the strengths and problems you identified, and the client-centered interview results.

Intervention Continuum

Adjunctive	**Enabling**	**Purposeful**	**Occupation-Based**
Interventions that prepare for performance and participation	*Interventions that focus on performance skills*	*Interventions that have a pre-determined goal and facilitate practice and problem solving*	*Interventions that are perceived as desirable, match individualized goals, and occur in appropriate context*

The next step is to categorize the interventions you identified in the Intervention Brainstorm activity according to the intervention continuum. Designate the category into which each intervention falls by labeling the interventions "A," "E," "P," or "O" to reflect them as adjunctive, enabling, purposeful, or occupation-based.

Client-Centered Interview Results

STEP 1: Ask *your* client to think about the occupations he or she performs during a typical day and provide three to five responses to the following:

Occupations client needs to do:

1.

2.

3.

4.

5.

Occupations client wants to do:

1.

2.

3.

4.

5.

Occupations client is expected to do:

1.

2.

3.

4.

5.

STEP 2: Ask *your* client to circle his or her five most important occupations.

Intervention Brainstorm

Make a list of interventions to include in *your* client's occupational therapy intervention plan based on his or her occupational profile and analysis of occupational performance, the strengths and problems you identified, and the client-centered interview results.

Intervention Continuum

Adjunctive	Enabling	Purposeful	Occupation-Based
Interventions that prepare for performance and participation	*Interventions that focus on performance skills*	*Interventions that have a pre-determined goal and facilitate practice and problem solving*	*Interventions that are perceived as desirable, match individualized goals, and occur in appropriate context*

The next step is to categorize the interventions you identified in the Intervention Brainstorm activity according to the intervention continuum. Designate the category into which each intervention falls by labeling the interventions "A," "E," "P," or "O" to reflect them as adjunctive, enabling, purposeful, or occupation-based.

Session Plan—Intervention Continuum

Identify one of your client's priority occupations:

Using interventions from the "Intervention Brainstorm," develop an occupational therapy session for *your* client.

A Adjunctive Interventions	**E** Enabling Interventions	**P** Purposeful Interventions	**O** Occupation-Based Interventions

Now develop a second occupational therapy session for the client. Consider progressing to the next session or to a session that is closer to discontinuation of occupational therapy intervention.

Identify which of *your* client's priority occupation(s) will be addressed in this session:

A Adjunctive Interventions	**E** Enabling Interventions	**P** Purposeful Interventions	**O** Occupation-Based Interventions

INDEX

INDEX

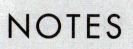

NOTES

NOTES

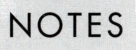

NOTES

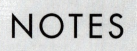

NOTES